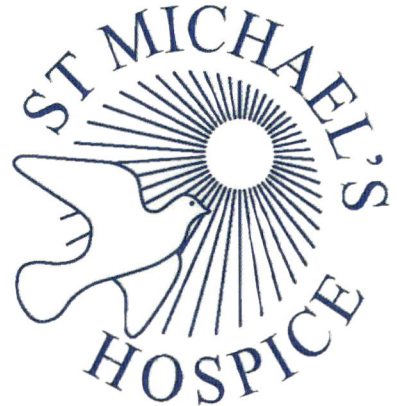

20 Beds - A Book of Life and Hope

First published in Great Britain in 2016 by A Way With Media Ltd, Shrewsbury, SY3 7LN, and
Hey Everyone Ltd, Hereford, HR2 6LR.

A CIP catalogue record for this book is available from the British Library.

ISBN - 9781910469019

Editor, publisher: Andy Richardson

Co-publishers: Andy Cooke, Rachel Haworth

Editorial production and layout design: David Briggs

Additional writing: Carl Jones

Printed and bound by 1010 Printing Group Ltd, China.

www.awaywithmedia.com

www.heyeveryone.com

CONTENTS

BUCKINGHAM PALACE
LONDON SW1A 1AA

It has been my honour and privilege to be involved with St Michael's Hospice in Herefordshire since its beginning in 1984.

During that time, hundreds of families have had reason to be grateful to the caring, compassionate team at St Michael's.

The high level of palliative care offered by its skilled staff and the tireless work done by community fundraisers to meet the ever-rising running costs is commendable.

St Michael's remains committed to providing quality care to those with progressive, life-limiting conditions, and to offer support to their families and carers too.

To all Staff Members, Volunteers and Friends of St Michael's Hospice I congratulate you on your 30th Anniversary and wish every success for the future expansion plans.

Alexandra

HRH Princess Alexandra

St Michael's Hospice – The story so far

Small beginnings, big ideas

Never underestimate people power. And never, ever tell a group of dedicated fundraisers that something cannot be achieved – because you can be sure they will pull out all the stops to prove you wrong!

St Michael's Hospice is a story of visionary triumph in the face of sometimes mountainous obstacles; a tale of faith, determination, perseverance, and the very essence of Britain's 'can-do' community spirit.

All spearheaded by a group of special, inspirational people whose legacy now stands proudly for all to see.

But let us begin at the very beginning.

Back in the 1970s, the concept of a hospice dedicated entirely to the provision of care for the sick and terminally ill, outside what was viewed as the 'traditional' hospital environment, was on relatively few people's radar.

These establishments, which were quietly beginning to crop up in various parts of the UK, placed the highest possible value on dignity, respect, and the wishes of both the patient and their families, and aimed to look after all their needs – be they medical, emotional, social, practical, psychological or spiritual.

But in the 1970s, there simply weren't too many of them around. And back then, people seemed to have an in-built suspicion of anything in the healthcare sector which was 'private', and which stood outside the rules, regulations and auspices of the National Health Service.

With hospices playing such a pivotal role in our communities these days, it's difficult to imagine how different things were back then. But it serves as a reminder of just how great a challenge the founders of St Michael's Hospice faced. And the magnitude of their achievements.

Before they could even start raising funds, these pioneers had to prove the need, and explain the hospice concept to those who would – they sincerely hoped – become committed to helping fund it for years to come.

Dr Richard Miller was one of the trailblazers. At the time, he was working as a GP in Hereford, and it was when he was looking after a patient, and very good friend, with advanced cancer, that the seeds of an idea were sown in his mind.

"Having been deeply involved throughout my friend's illness from diagnosis to his subsequent death, I was acutely aware of the devastating effects the disease had on him and his young family," he recalls.

"I was equally aware of the gaps in my knowledge of the control of distressing symptoms, and my feelings of inadequacy when dealing with death and bereavement."

All of this was compounded by a lack of suitable facilities in the Herefordshire area which he felt could help.

"Back then, people were mostly looked after in hospital, or at home. There was little understanding of symptom control, and

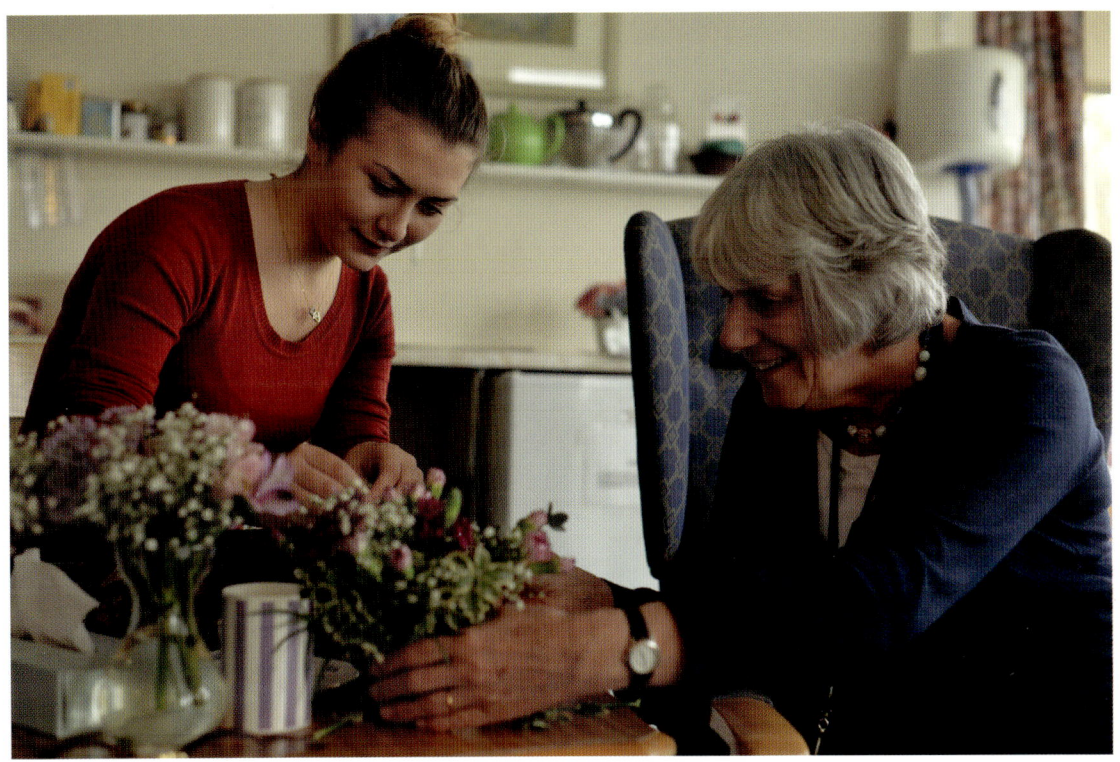

people often died in pain, screened off in the corner. I, along with other health care professionals, found this very difficult to deal with."

Richard adds: "My wife and I visited a number of hospices around the UK and were deeply impressed by the very special atmosphere in each of the units, and the outstanding care given – not just to the patients, but to their families.

"I was very keen to improve my skills in the care of dying and, for the next three years, I spent all my study leave working in hospices."

It was while at St Barnabas Hospice in Worthing that Richard came under the spell of Dr Francis Gusterson, known to everyone as Gus. The former anaesthetist had founded the centre and, along with Dame Cicely Saunders, was one of the pioneers of the modern hospice movement.

Gus, who remained hugely supportive of St Michael's throughout its early years, was passionate in sharing his knowledge of, and enormous enthusiasm for hospice care, and the time which Richard spent at St Barnabas Hospice merely cemented his view that such a facility was desperately needed in Herefordshire.

But Richard was acutely aware that this was not something he could achieve on his own.

Little did he know that another like-minded campaigner was about to enter his life.

It was in 1979 that Richard first encountered the diminutive dynamo called Freda Pearce, whose team had just completed an impressive and hugely efficient appeal to raise £90,000 for a body scanner at Cheltenham General

Hospital.

As luck would have it, she was about to embark on her next fundraising marathon . . . to build a hospice in Herefordshire!

The morning after he heard of Freda's plans, Richard found himself on her doorstep. He remembers: "I introduced myself and informed her that we shared a common ambition.

"The effect was electric; in no time at all Freda was planning a fundraising campaign and using her existing group as a base, a number of potentially interested people were approached and a fundraising and planning committee was formed.

"The Hospice appeal was launched just a few weeks later, and there was immediate interest and enthusiasm locally. That has never changed; the support of the general public has remained amazing, and been our main source of income."

The third pivotal member of that founding team back then was another local medic, Dr Jeff Kramer.

A Londoner who had worked at high-profile hospitals including Great Ormond Street, he had moved up to Hereford in 1970 to become the hospital's first ever consultant haematologist.

He says: "I remember coming out of the hospital one day and chatting with Richard, who told me about the meeting he had had with Freda, and the ideas which were beginning to take shape.

"What did I think about the idea of helping to establish a hospice? he asked me.

"Well, I'd seen how terminally ill patients often languished in hospital wards for the last two or three weeks of their lives. Nursing staff did their best to keep them comfortable, but they were rushed off their feet with other duties, and it was a far from ideal situation."

And so, Jeff attended a meeting, held in the front room of Dr Richard Miller's home, with Freda Pearce and a handful of other keen volunteers also in attendance.

"I've got to be honest, I did have my doubts about whether we would ever be able to raise enough cash," he admits.

"We had calculated that we would need about £750,000 just to get the Hospice physically built – but that was just the start. Then we had to find enough money on top of that to keep it running.

"It was pure faith and a belief in the project being the right thing to do that gave us the will to go on.

"Freda led the team of fundraisers; she had the cheek of the devil and was a very powerful person. She believed nothing was impossible, and through sheer dedication and love for our fellow men and women, we succeeded.

"I remember Freda cadging a lift from me on the way home from that first meeting at Richard's house; that was when we had a good old chat and a laugh and got to know one another for the first time.

"It was clear from that moment that this determined woman was the perfect person to drive the fundraising forward. She refused to accept that anything was impossible."

Further regular meetings were held, often at the Conservative Club in West Street, Hereford, and a plan of action began to take shape. Freda's foundation would front the fundraising effort, and a second, separate committee would be created to handle operational affairs.

Among those playing pivotal roles at this time were fellow founders including Rev John Hall-Matthews, Peter Hill, and Sandra Griffiths – whose many fundraising achievements including founding and

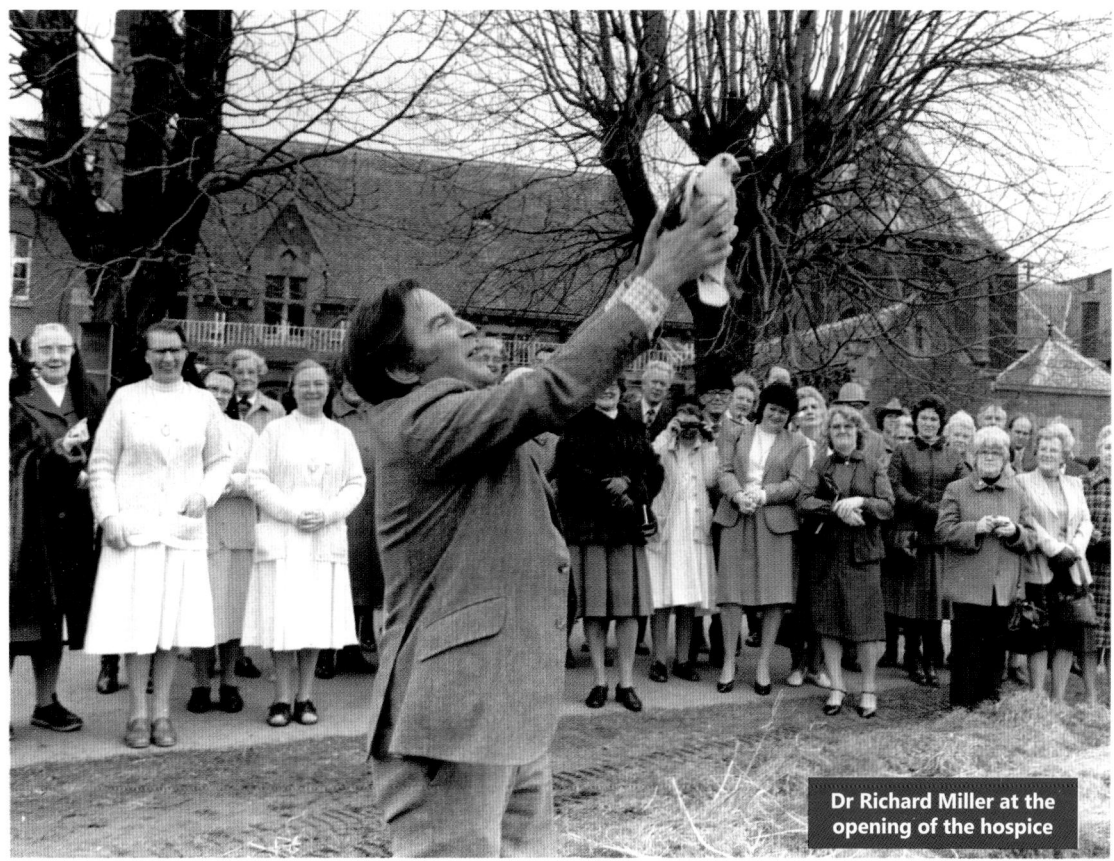

Dr Richard Miller at the opening of the hospice

launching the annual Hereford Marathon.

Another of the original members at that initial meeting in Richard's home, who would go on to play a pivotal role in the Hospice story for three decades, was Olwyn Barnett.

She was, in the words of local journalist Bill Tanner, recognised as a redoubtable – often indefatigable – opponent in the local council chamber, who transferred that same tenacity to causes behind the scenes, particularly in the areas of education and social care.

Olwyn was struck by cancer herself on more than one occasion, and ended up seeing hospice life from the other side, when she spent time at St Michael's as an in-patient, shortly before passing away peacefully at home in November 2014.

She had received her 35 year Long Service award the previous year, while at the Hospice, and looked back fondly at those early days, and what had been achieved since.

"I think it's fair to say we were all 'trapped' by this little lady called Freda Pearce. Everyone thought we were pretty mad, or bloody-minded I suppose, but we managed to gel into a team.

"Thirty years on, the dream is far more than a reality. We were helped, of course, by all of the areas – particularly from my point of view, over in Powys. Places like Presteigne, Knighton, Kington, Llandrindod Wells were all so supportive.

"We used to take Freda out there in the early days. She captured the imagination of people; she was very, very good, and very few people failed to help her.

"There is a feeling that everyone who has contributed to St Michael's feels part and parcel of it, and I think that this was a very important thing we did in the early days. We made people realise it was their Hospice."

When Olwyn's cancer returned for a final time, though, she checked into the Hospice as an in-patient, because she said she felt 'totally out of control with it'.

She summed up her experience at St Michael's as 'a privilege'.

"I was asked whether I would like to come in, and I have to say it was a privilege for me to see at first-hand what is done, and to have benefited from what is done."

When Olwyn was appointed chairman of Herefordshire Council in her final years, she started an appeal for St Michael's, pledging to raise 'a great deal of money'.

"Out there, there are more people like Freda – too many to mention by name – waiting in the wings to do what we did in the very beginning.

"They are all there. They have different names, but let's get to it. In other words, me being my usual direct self, could we please get up off our backsides and start all over again, and go the extra mile."

Jeff Kramer remembers Olwyn's can-do attitude for the Hospice as legendary: "She was fantastically energetic with a great basic wisdom. An amazing, formidable lady through her outlook and enthusiasm, she got things done and was always so supportive of the Hospice and the people who worked for it."

It was Olwyn's dying wish that the Hospice hold an event which mirrored some of the

Freda Pearce MBE

Freda Kathleen Pearce was born on October 3, 1912 in a small mining community called Leeswood, near Mold in north east Wales.

With her father working down the mines, and her mother wheelchair-bound, she left school at the age of 13 to look after her seven brothers and sisters.

Her childhood was a largely happy time, although she would recall that it was only thanks to the local soup kitchens that her family was able to keep food on the table during the testing times of the General Strike in 1926.

At the age of 18, Freda left home and went into service as a Lady's companion, and three years later, she found herself in Hereford for the first time in another caring role, this time looking after a sick aunt.

It was here that she met the man who would become her husband, local police officer Vic Pearce, and the couple settled in the area and had two children, Vic and Pat.

Freda took a job as an assistant buyer at Greenlands department store, as well as being appointed chief children's buyer at Lindsey Price

Sadly, her husband Vic didn't enjoy good health, and Freda gave up work to devote herself to caring for him during the last 30 years of his life. Vic died in 1983.

For the final decade of her husband's life, Freda had not been in the greatest of health herself. In 1974 she was diagnosed with cervical cancer

ethos and spirit of the original fundraising events, stimulating fundraisers for the future in the way that the original Freda Pearce ladies did, and engaging those original ladies for one more time. And so, Elaine Furber and

– the woman behind the legend

nd underwent an intensive programme of adiotherapy.

The prognosis was not good. When she was ischarged from hospital, she was given just six onths to live.

But, however long she had left, Freda vowed use her time to good purpose, and set about aising funds for the purchase of a body scanner. he told her daughter Pat: "God touched me and et me the work to do."

With the help of an enthusiastic committee, an stonishing £178,000 was raised and Freda had he honour of being presented to The Princess oyal, Princess Anne.

She'd been bitten by the fundraising bug and ext on her agenda was the idea of starting a ospice for Herefordshire.

In 1979, the Freda Pearce Foundation was ormed, and was instrumental in raising the cash build St Michael's Hospice.

No potential donor was off limits to Freda – she ven secured a £50,000 donation from the King of audi Arabia!

The Queen recognised Freda's tireless undraising by awarding her the MBE in 1982, nd inviting her to a royal garden party.

But she refused to take all the plaudits, nsisting that she only ever received the honour ecause of the generosity of the public, and the edication of her fellow workers.

Sadly, the seemingly indomitable Freda

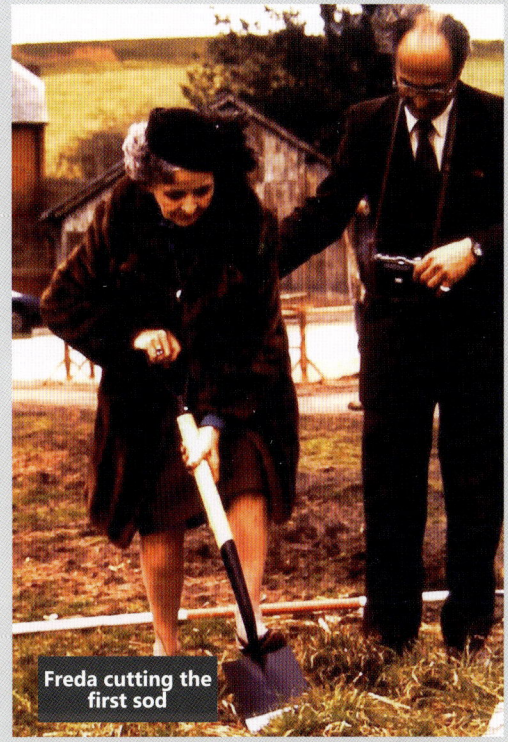

Freda cutting the first sod

Pearce never got the chance to see her St Michael's Hospice dream become a reality, as she died in 1983 shortly before building work was completed.

But her legacy lives on. Special permission was granted for Freda to be buried just a stone's throw from the Hospice, in the grounds of the neighbouring convent.

Mary Thomas – two of the originals – threw themselves with typical gusto into helping organise a Christmas Fair, helped by some of the longest-serving Hospice staff, and Olwyn's daughter Debbie.

That family atmosphere at St Michael's – with staff and volunteers rallying to every cause, and responding to the needs of each other – was to become a recurring theme over the years.

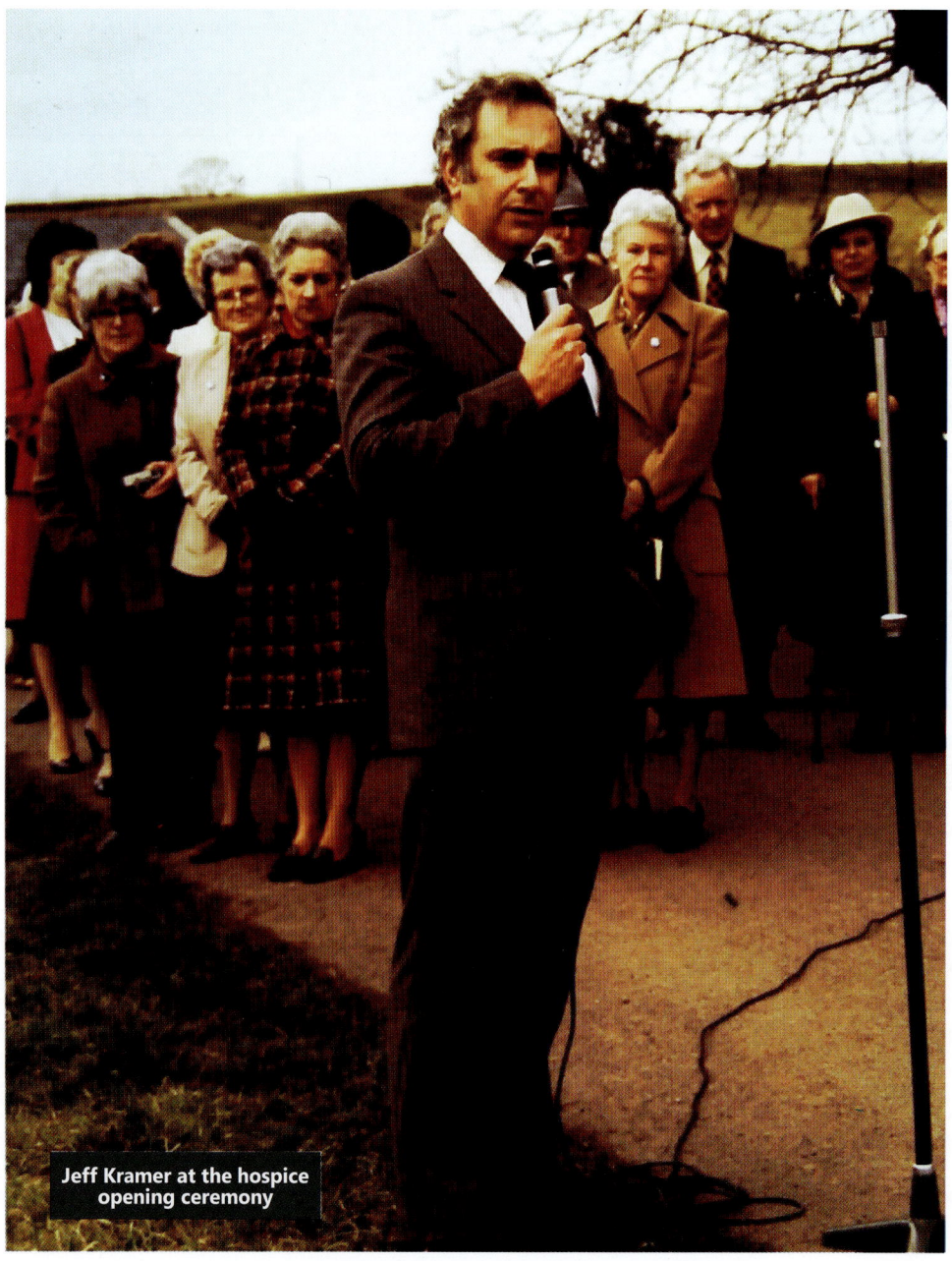

Jeff Kramer at the hospice opening ceremony

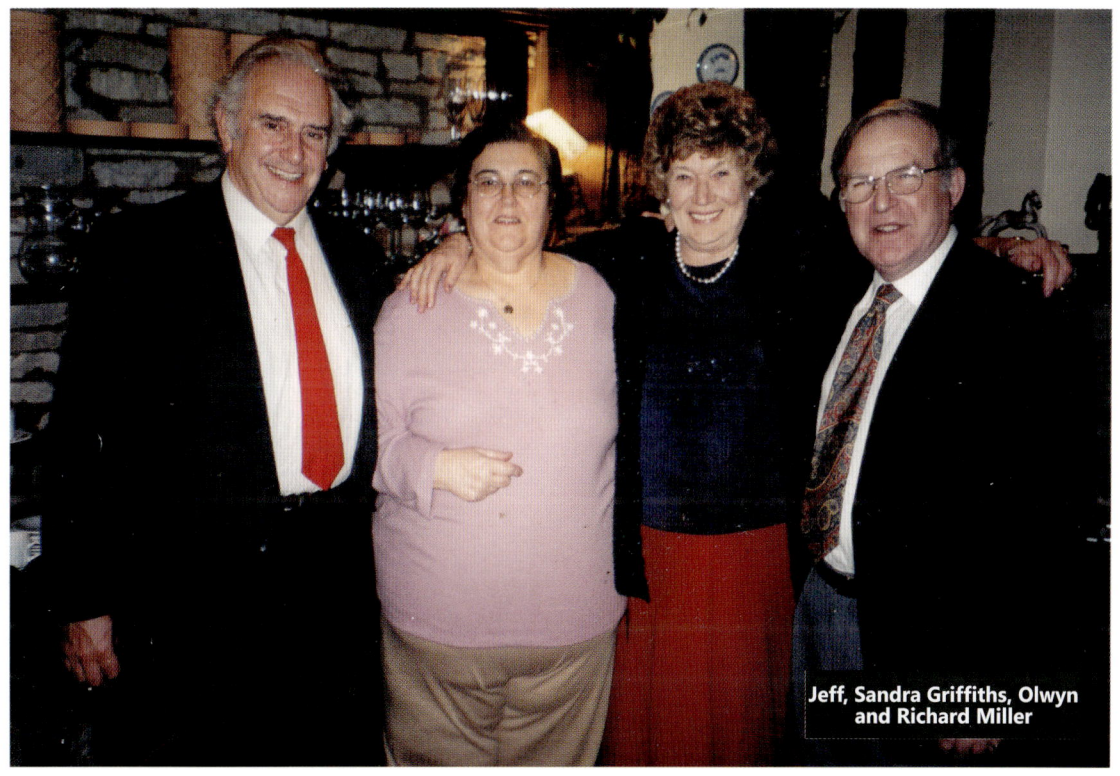

Jeff, Sandra Griffiths, Olwyn and Richard Miller

Finding the right location

So, the need was established, the nucleus of a campaign committee was in place, but one key question remained unanswered. Where could this new Hospice be built?

It needed to be a site which was reasonably close to the centre of Hereford, in a tranquil setting sympathetic to patient needs, convenient for commuting visitors . . . but most importantly of all, available, and at the right price!

The fundraising team visited many locations within a 10-mile radius of Hereford city centre, one of which was Bartestree Convent, a few miles from Hereford city centre on the road to Ledbury.

The Convent of Our Lady of Charity & Refuge was founded in 1863 and for decades the imposing red brick building received girls who had been placed into the convent's care by local authorities.

Richard Miller remembers: "We received a wonderful welcome from the sisters who gave us a fascinating tour of the convent and its grounds.

"Just as we were starting to think that none of it was going to be quite suitable for our needs, we found ourselves in a small orchard to the rear of the building.

"We were greatly moved by the serenity of the place and its amazing view. It seemed the ideal site for our Hospice."

From that moment on, every other potential venue was held up against the Bartestree benchmark, and they all fell short.

And so, negotiations with the Convent owners began in earnest.

Very quickly, it was agreed that the Hospice committee could lease the land from the sisters for a peppercorn rent of just 5p a year, for 99 years.

The Hospice committee would enjoy a very warm relationship with the sisters until they were sadly forced to leave in 1992 when the Convent lost its referral contract from Herefordshire County Council.

Liverpool-based development firm Millfield subsequently won planning permission to convert the building into a hall of residence for students, and build more than 40 homes on the orchard in front of the convent.

It could have been a tricky situation for St Michael's, but the developers were happy to gift the land on which the Hospice stands – along with a derelict cottage close by – to the board, meaning they would hold the freehold of the land for the first time.

Olwyn Barnett said: "The board of directors were very appreciative of this very generous gift, which certainly helped secure the Hospice's long-term future."

Site secured . . . now to raise the funds.

Building a hospice from a standing start is a long, painstaking, and expensive task, requiring meticulous organisation and unswerving dedication.

In those first few months, The Freda Pearce Foundation – which already had its infrastructure in place having raised funds for the body scanner in Cheltenham – took the lead.

It was this foundation which was instrumental in raising more than £350,000 to get the project under way.

Their contribution was not lost on HRH Princess Alexandra when she arrived to perform the official opening of St Michael's –

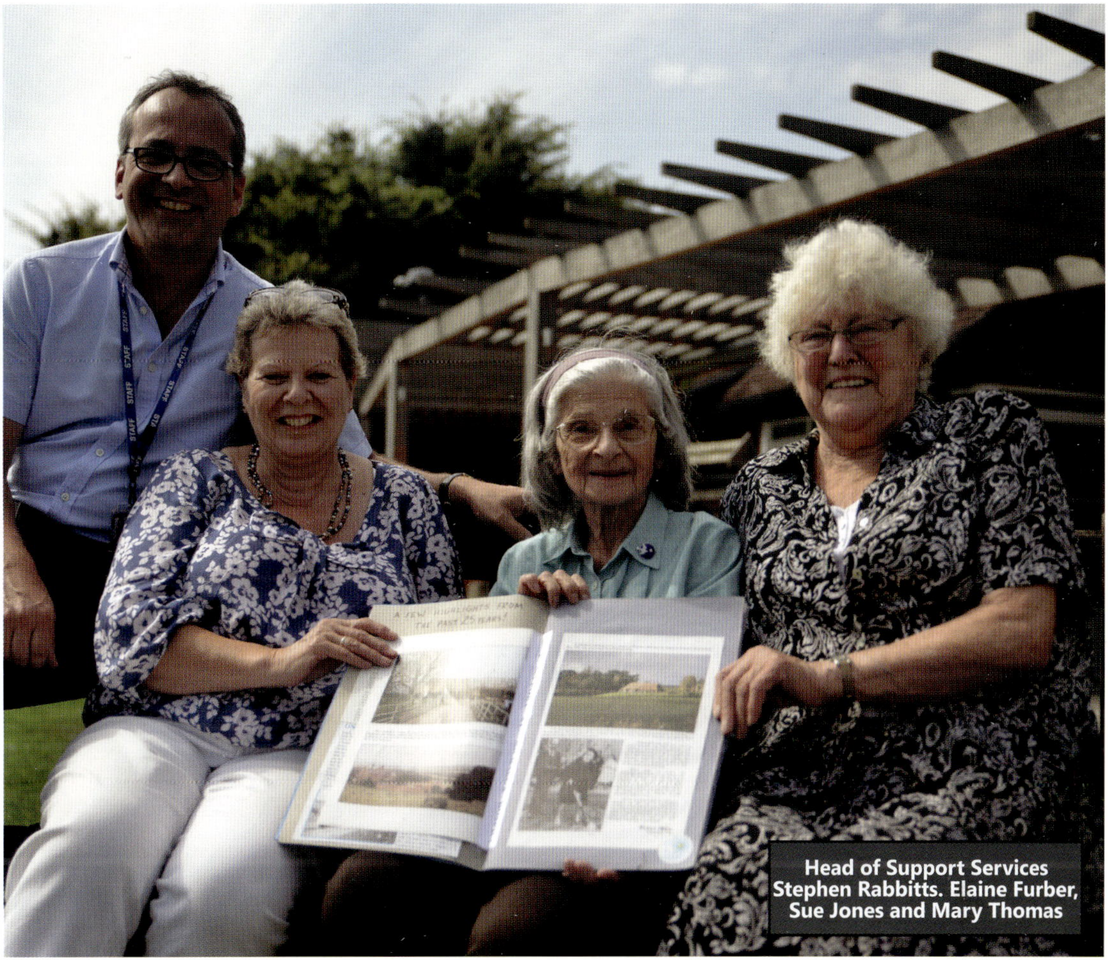

Head of Support Services
Stephen Rabbitts. Elaine Furber,
Sue Jones and Mary Thomas

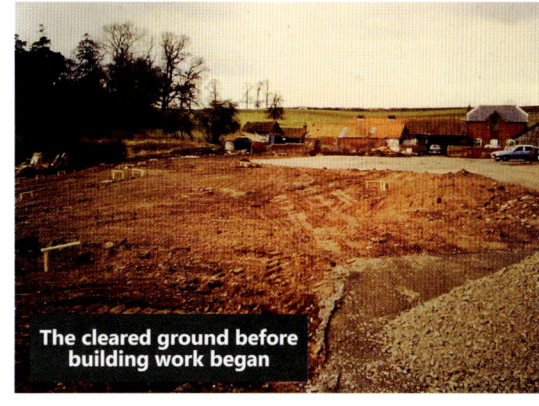

The cleared ground before
building work began

she would not go to lunch until she had been officially introduced to 'Freda's Ladies' that she had heard so much about! Word of their achievements had clearly percolated Royal circles.

Herefordshire Amateur Rafters also played an important part at this time, agreeing to help raise funds for one of the wards. In 1980 they amassed £10,000 from a host of events, and fared even better the following year, adding a further £15,000 to the coffers.

It was a logical step for Tricia Hales, chairman of the rafters, to subsequently join The Freda Pearce Foundation, sitting on its executive committee and fundraising group and helping to found the Freda Pearce League of Friends in 1985, which continued its tireless fundraising work.

Everywhere, across towns, villages and hamlets in the area, people were doing their bit to support the hospice campaign. Things were rapidly gathering momentum.

One particular group of friends – Dorothy Stainton, Arthur and Freda Woodward, Betty and Jack Swaithes and Eric Bayliss – got together to hold a whist drive in August 1985, which raised an amazing £4,260. But that was just the start…

When the local newspaper revealed the Hospice was having trouble funding some of its nurses, the group set up a standing order to subsidise the wage bill; a system which continued for many years.

In 1998, the group was granted charitable status and is now known as the Eric Bayliss Fund for St Michael's Hospice. It raised a staggering £150,000 in the hospice's first 20 years, and still donates £1,250 per month to pay towards a nurse's salary.

But back in early 1982, the fundraising committee was still a long, long way short of the initial £750,000 required to build their St Michael's dream.

On July 1st 1982, the committee convened to formulate an action plan, and it was here that Jeff Kramer made a crucial move; without which, it is no exaggeration to say, the Hospice might never have been built.

He contacted Sir James Ackers, the maverick Midlands businessman who at that time had not long taken over at the helm of the West Midlands Regional Health Authority

"I had heard that the Regional Health Authority had given grants to other places in the West Midlands, so I thought nothing ventured, nothing gained.

"I wrote to Sir James, outlining our financial position and asking if the Authority would be in a position to provide us with a similar grant to help our cause.

"He got back to me and said that, unfortunately, he was not able to give us a grant – but revealed that the Authority would instead be prepared to provide us with a £400,000 interest-free loan.

"Well, I thought, that's better than a kick in the pants! It would make up the shortfall in our fundraising, and mean we could go ahead with confidence, employing architects, and starting to build the Hospice.

"I'm not sure it is true to say that the Hospice would never have been built without that loan, but it would certainly have taken us several years longer to raise the money without it."

With this loan in their clutches to supplement the fruits of the not insignificant local fundraising efforts, the committee set about finding a builder, appointing local firm H Vaughan & Sons.

A Herefordshire architect, Nigel Dees, had been deeply involved with the Hospice committee from the outset, and so was the obvious choice to draw up the plans.

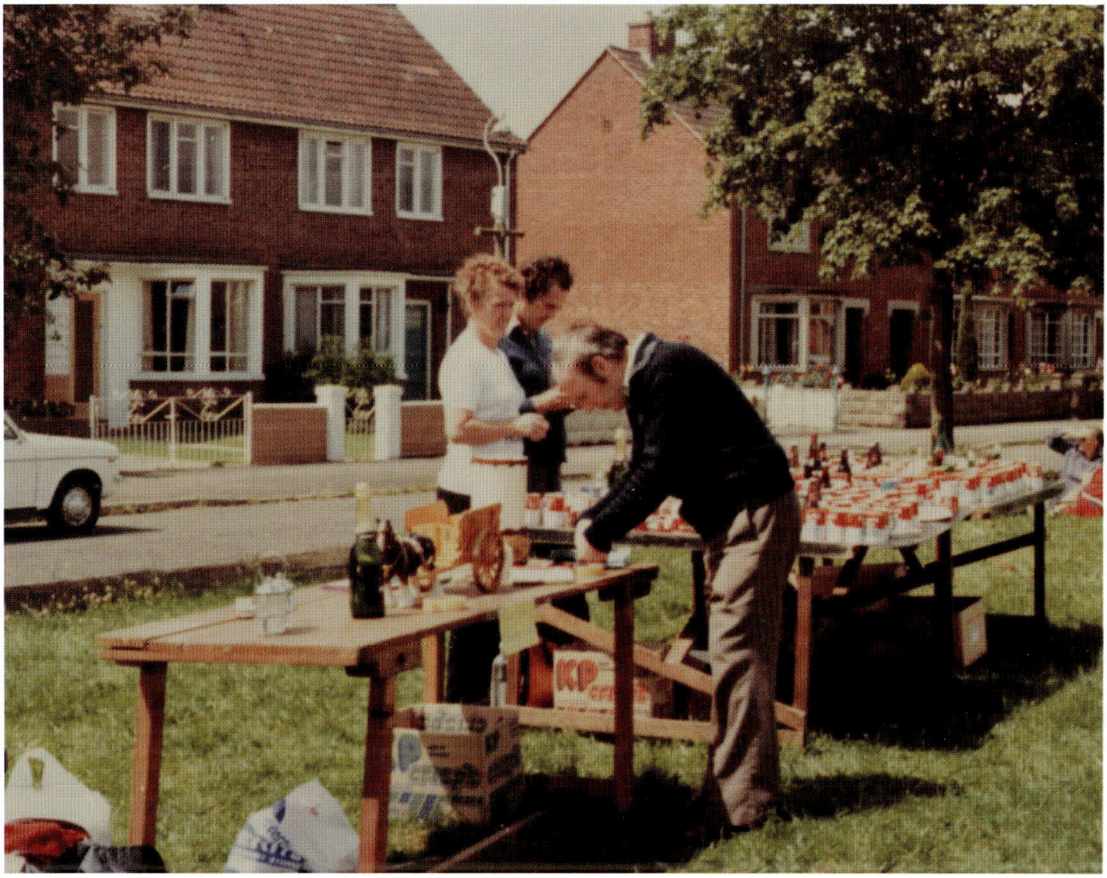

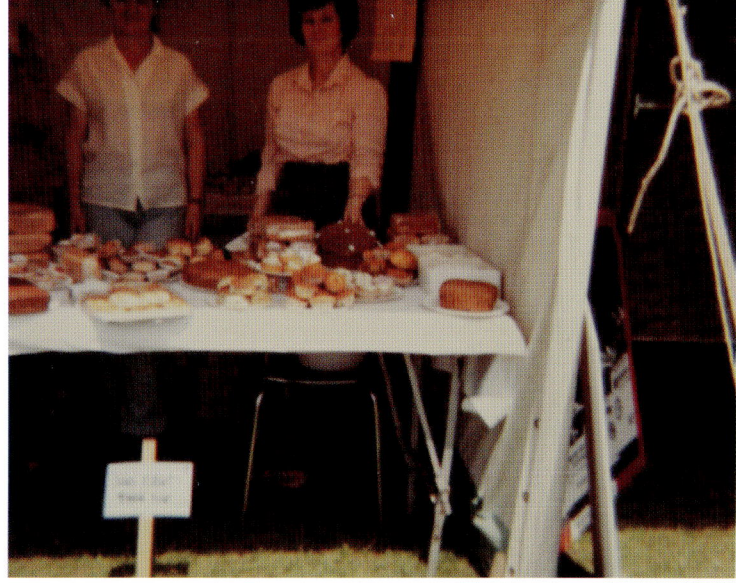

Raising funds was an ongoing challenge for the hospice in its early years

It was a task he embraced with relish, spending time visiting a number of similar sites around the country to seek inspiration.

Nigel incorporated many of the best aspects he had gleaned, and worked closely with surveyor Brian Adams to produce a plan for the attractive, innovative building which made best use of the site, giving patients the benefit of the magnificent views of the countryside.

The building was completed in the summer of 1984, at a total cost of three quarters of a million pounds, and St Michael's proudly admitted its first patient on October 31, 1984.

Her Royal Highness Princess Alexandra performed the official opening in May 1985 – and Jeff Kramer had an encounter with the VIP visitor that day which still brings a smile to his face.

"The Princess was being introduced to the management team and was eager to find out more about how we had raised money to build it. I was first in line to tell her about the Hospice, and she asked me 'Are you well endowed?'. Well, I must admit, I blushed! I said something like 'It's early days yet, ma'am'.

"I know she was referring to our finances, but the way it came out was just so funny. Everyone had a laugh about it . . . including the Princess when she realised what she had said."

A local journalist had overheard the conversation, and one way or another, the light-hearted royal faux-pas found its way into the Nigel Dempster column in the Daily Mail the following day!

And so, with a mixture of pride, emotion and relief, St Michael's Hospice had been built, and officially launched. The dream had become a bricks and mortar reality.

In many ways, though, the hard work was only just beginning – the committee now had to find sufficient funds to run and maintain it.

What's in a name?

It was agreed, quite early on in the planning stages, that the Hospice's name needed to reflect the important spiritual dimension in the planning and day-to-day running of the operation.

St Michael was felt to be particularly appropriate as he represents the eventual triumph of good over evil, and is said to accompany the dying on their final journey.

He is mentioned five times in the Old Testament. Daniel 12:1 says: "At that time there shall arise Michael, the great prince, guardian of your people."

There is also a local community back story to the St Michael's Hospice logo.

The committee approached Hereford College of Art to see if a group of the students would take up the challenge to design a logo.

They did so with relish, and Jane Cross produced an inspiring design which captured the essence of the Hospice's philosophy, depicting the Dove of Peace flying into the Light.

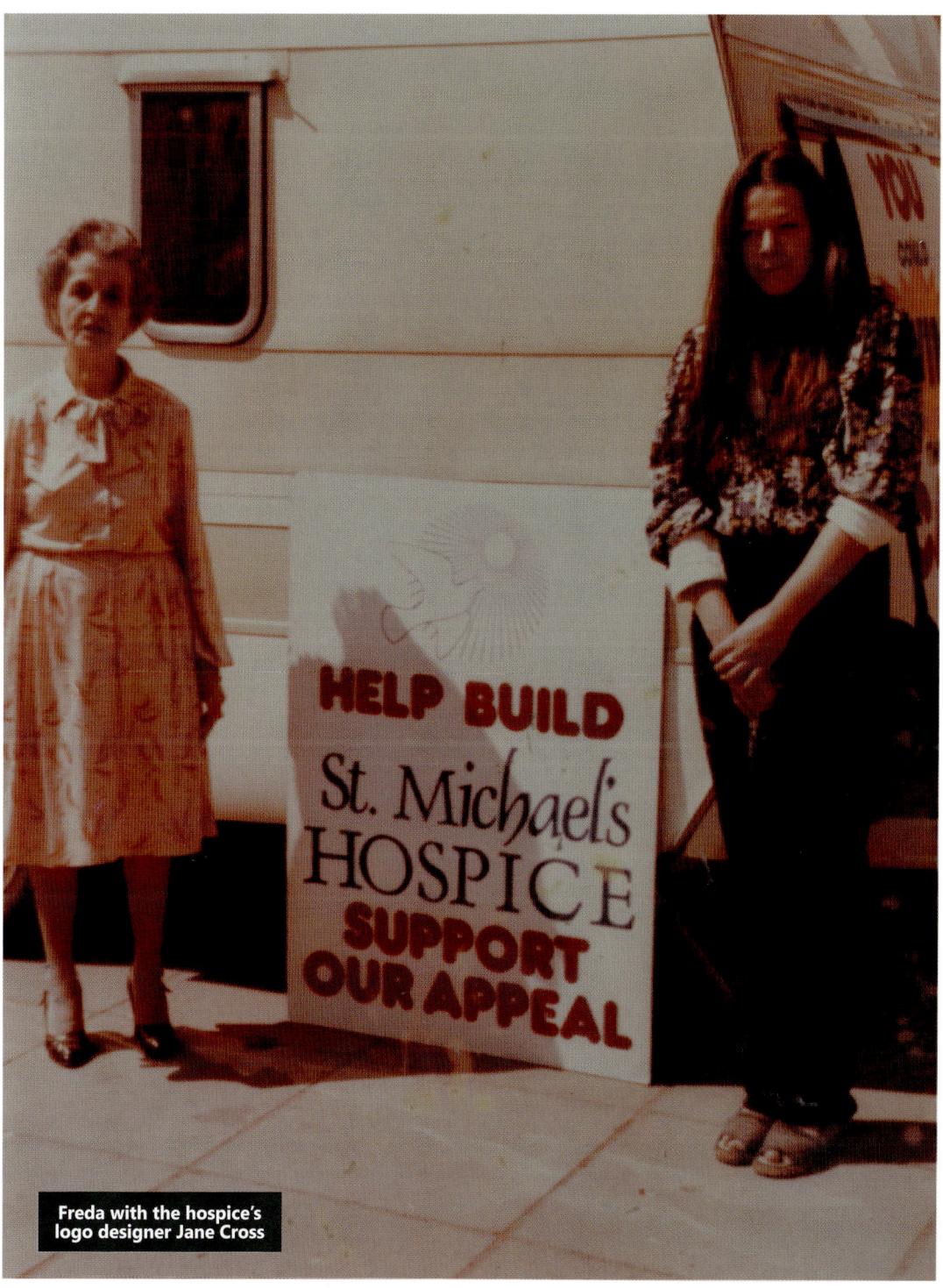

Freda with the hospice's
logo designer Jane Cross

Riding the rollercoaster

Although only five years had passed between that first exploratory meeting with Freda, and the Hospice opening, it had been far from plain sailing.

Aside from the daunting task of raising the money to construct and run the building, the committee had encountered considerable opposition from some fairly influential people.

Richard Miller recalls: "A leading, and highly respected member of the Hospice movement, tried very hard to persuade us to start with just a Home Care facility.

"I am convinced that, had we done this, Herefordshire would have been waiting for its hospice to be built for at least another 20 years, as happened in other parts of the country. Our determination to have an in-patient unit never wavered – and we were proved right."

There were some difficult personnel issues in those first few years, though, which brought unwelcome media attention to the Hospice.

Matrons and clinical directors came and went as the committee battled to find the right blend of compassion, flexibility and business acumen among its fledgling management team.

Dame Margaret Shepherd, who had played an integral and leading role on the committee in the founding years and was President of the Council of Management at the time of this period of flux, stepped down as president of the Freda Pearce Foundation in 1986.

There are differing accounts about what exactly caused the situation, and whilst the media were quick to pick up on possible contentions within the Hospice ranks, including in an editorial comment column in the Hereford Times on June 5, Trustee and founding Hospice member Dr Jeffrey Kramer recalls: "I admired Dame Margaret greatly when I was the first chairman of the Council of Management (as it was called in those days) and she was our President, which we regarded as our highest honour...There was really no excessive discord or argument, but full and thorough debates."

As the editorial in the Hereford Times concluded: "There can only be one objective – the growing from strength to strength of the unit – the dream of the late Freda Pearce who inspired such support from the public. That spirit must be rekindled."

It was. This short period of adverse publicity, which , it must be acknowledged does not concur with other accounts of the same time period about what was going on behind the scenes at the Hospice, proved to be something of a watershed for St Michaels, which had been on a steep, and very public learning curve over those first couple of years.

Personnel problems soon passed as the team knitted together, backed by representatives of some major local businesses and a growing army of loyal volunteers. Giles Bulmer, a prominent member of the cider-making Bulmer family, played an important role in getting the Hospice on a businesslike footing. He chaired the Development Trust for a time, and remained a trustee for many years.

"I use an RAF analogy to describe those early months," Jeff Kramer says. "We took off quickly, hit a bit of turbulence in our first ascent, but continued to gain height and

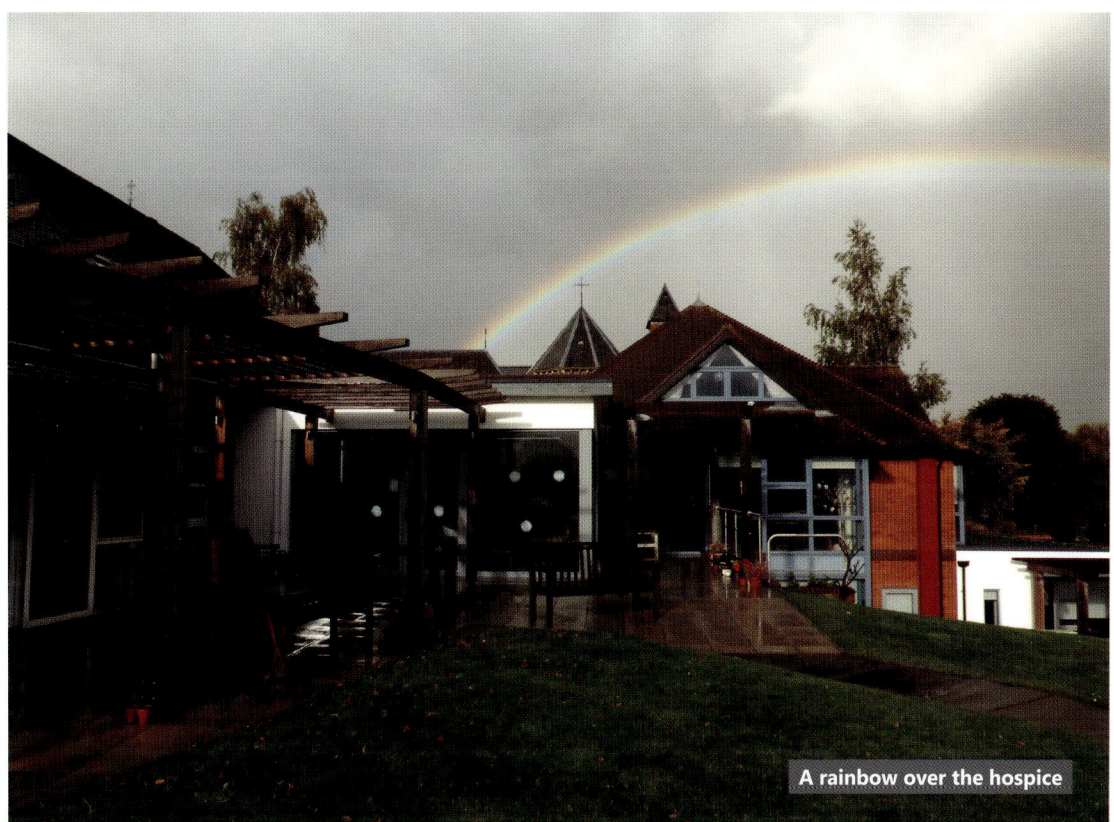

A rainbow over the hospice

eventually stabilised."

The only battles the team continued to face revolved around keeping sufficient funds coming in to enable the Hospice to continue on a safe financial footing.

Olwyn Barnett, who chaired the board in those early years, recalled the tough financial times, in a speech she delivered during the 10th anniversary year.

"Ever since the building was completed, the Hospice has had a bumpy financial ride," she declared. "There has never been a time when fundraisers have been able to sit back and rest on their laurels.

"We are proud of the service that has been

given to over 2,000 patients and their families in the 10 years since St Michael's was opened. The care and compassion shown by staff and volunteers cannot be measured."

The Hospice also benefited from some incredibly generous bequests. One which made headlines in those early years was a timely Christmas gift at the end of 1986, when Malvern musician Jane Parke left £60,000 in her will. There were many, many more just like it.

On Saturday September 17, 1994, all six bell towers in Hereford rang out to celebrate the 10th anniversary of St Michael's Hospice.

In what turned out to be a marathon effort,

two teams of bellringers were led by head of nursing Jane Mason, and Chaplain David Bowen.

Between them, travelling in two minibuses kindly donated by South Herefordshire Garage for the day, they rang bells in more than 50 different church towers in one day – starting shortly after sunrise, and finishing at 9pm.

For the first decade, St Michael's had supplemented its in-patient activities by operating a Day Hospice in a room on the ground floor. By the mid 1990s, it became apparent that bigger and better facilities were needed.

Two become one

/ / Oh no, I couldn't possibly do that." That was Elizabeth Drew's reaction when she rebutted an initial approach in 1996 to chair the appeal to raise funds for a new Day Hospice.

John Caiger, from the then St Michael's Hospice Development Trust, asked her why.

"No-one knows me. I've never done anything like this before."

Well, you know what they say about taking a leap of faith? Elizabeth was eventually persuaded into taking on the challenge, and it turned out to be a wise decision for everyone concerned.

In less than 18 months, she and her committee – running what would go on to be christened the Sunflower Appeal – had raised the £600,000 required to see the project completed.

A purpose-built three-storey Day Hospice including a suite of rooms for meetings, offices, as well as a hair and beauty salon, was added to the existing Hospice.

Writing in the St Michael's 20th anniversary magazine, Elizabeth recalled the launch.

"It was held in College Hall, Hereford Cathedral, on June 14th 1996 – a beautiful, sunny day. We already had nearly £200,000 in the kitty and were thrilled when Viscount Portman surprised us all with a donation of £35,000."

The first sod was cut for the new Day Centre in August 1996 and the building was completed and in use by the following June. Princess Alexandra, who had performed the official opening of the first Hospice building back in May 1995, returned on July 29, 1997 to do the honours once again.

The success of the Sunflower Appeal meant that, each and every week, 70 people and their families could be cared for, monitored and given symptom control.

To many, this was a priceless, precious lifeline which allowed them to stay in their own homes for a longer time.

But attending Day Hospice is also a social occasion filled with fun, laughter, and a busy programme of activities.

"People never want to come here, and then they never want to leave," says former Day Hospice Sister, Hazel Brooke.

By this time, the Rev Preb Carl Attwood was chairman of St Michael's board of trustees. He went on to hold the chairmanship for a decade, from 1995 to 2005, and it was during his stewardship that the Hospice as a fully functioning business model really came of age.

He recalls: "I was already aware of the Hospice, of course, through my role as a

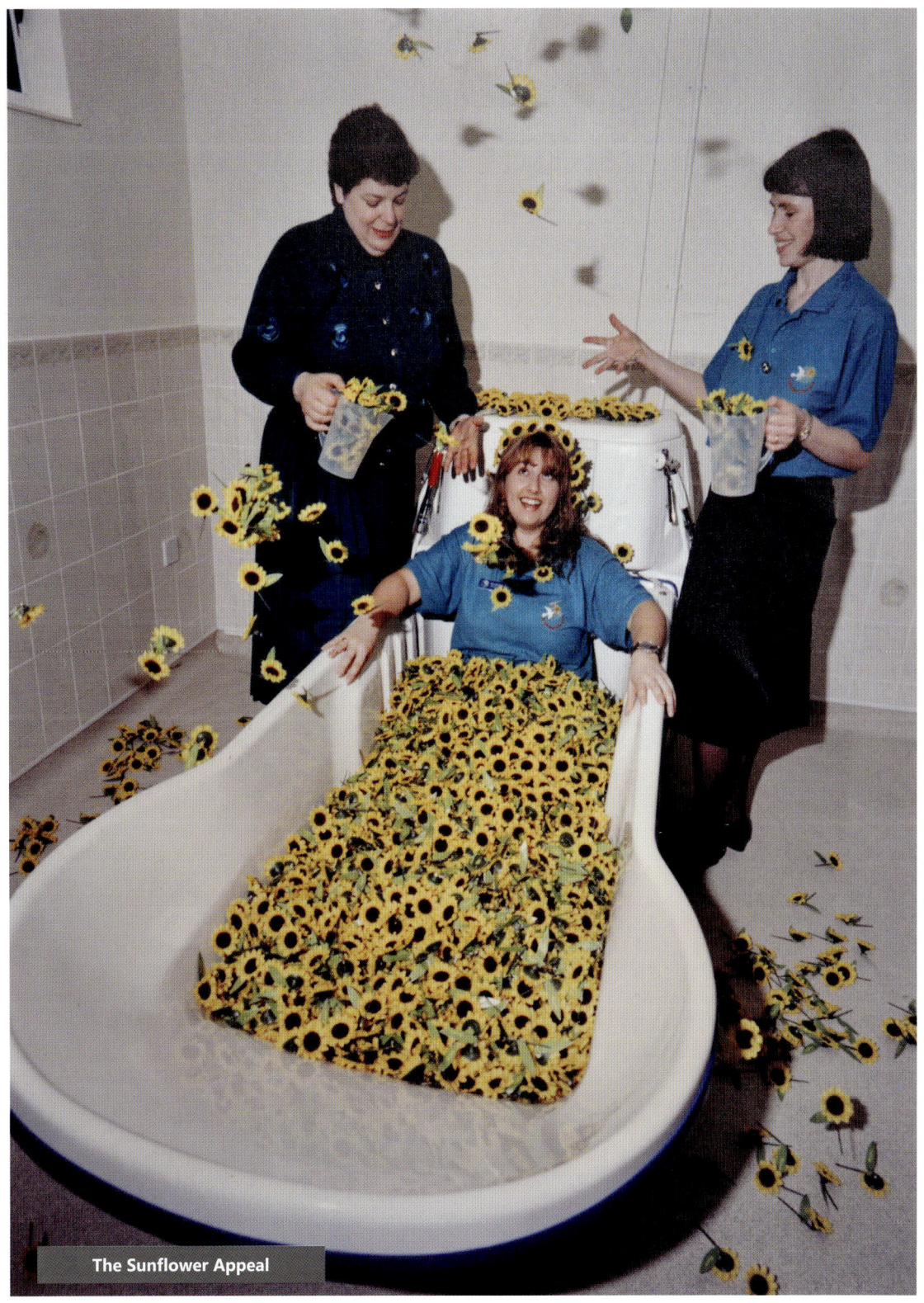

The Sunflower Appeal

local priest, but was made chairman very soon after being invited onto the board, with the task of overseeing a quite significant transition.

"When I arrived, the Hospice was split into two very distinctive areas; one dealing with fundraising, and one which was solely dedicated to the operational side of running the Hospice.

"It was very much a personality-led organisation, spearheaded of course by that pocket dynamo, Freda Pearce, who simply didn't know the meaning of the word 'no'.

"But times were changing. The sheer growth of the Hospice organisation since its creation, coupled with the rapidly increasing amount of rules and regulations which had to be complied with, meant the need for a change of focus."

Carl, who had been introduced to St Michael's by Jeff Kramer, was asked to write a paper, outlining what kind of restructuring programme he felt was needed.

"The two operational and fundraising divisions needed to be fully integrated, in my opinion, and I knew that this process could turn out to be quite a tricky and painful one. It's fair to say that some people were a bit nervous about what lay ahead.

"In the event, though, it was not too difficult at all. Yes, some people went, and some new faces were brought in to provide a different kind of perspective and slightly different blend of skills – that was always going to be inevitable.

"But considering we essentially changed the Hospice from a relatively small community-based structure to something which operated on much more formal business lines, I don't think the transition could have gone much better."

Carl recalls his job at that time as being a combination of 'delicate people-management, analysis and strategy', backed up by a 'stunning' executive team including the likes of Wyevale Garden Centres chairman Brian Evans, financial guru Roger Gates, and the aforementioned Elizabeth Drew, whose administrative skills were, in Carl's opinion, 'simply terrific'.

"The very essence of St Michael's Hospice – the reason it has such a special atmosphere – is that no one person is more important than anyone else.

"People are not there just because they are paid to be there; they are at the Hospice because they want to be there.

"While it was important to be running on more professional business lines going forward, what really set it apart – and continues to do so – is that it remains embedded in the voluntary community."

Carl continues: "For those who began the process all those years ago, the climate was very different. Hospices were in their infancy and there was a strong resistance in some areas to the whole idea of a service being led by 'amateurs'.

"The tenacity and determination of those first volunteers – many of whom have continued giving active support to the Hospice – in pursuing and achieving their dream is impressive and humbling."

During Carl's stewardship, the Hospice also had to contend with falling support from the Government.

Between the years of 1998 and 2003, the contribution towards running costs from the National Health Service reduced from 25% to around 19%, placing an ever-increasing burden on Herefordshire communities and the Hospice's own fundraising efforts.

A network of Hospice shops began to grow, and a lottery was launched. In 2001,

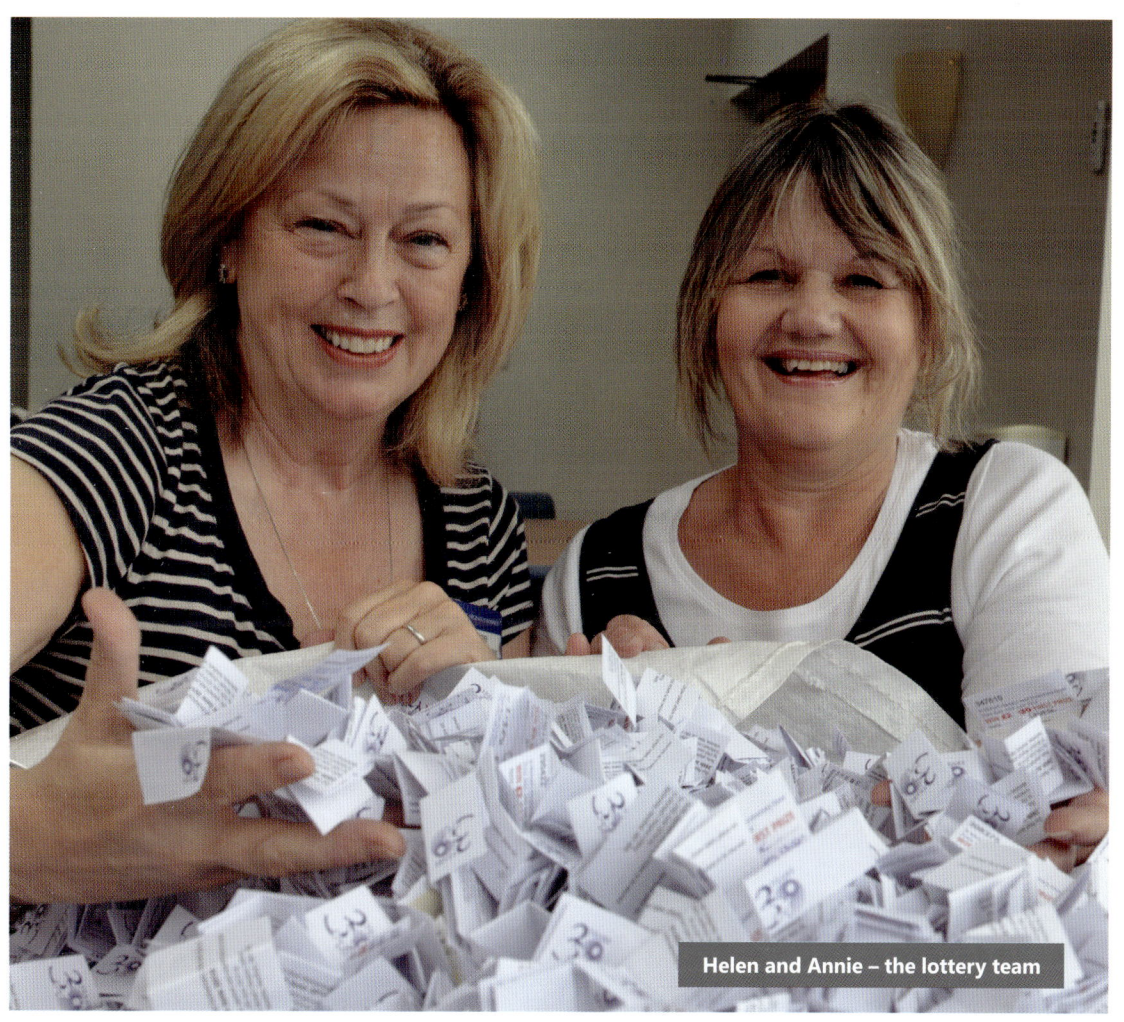

Helen and Annie – the lottery team

St Michael's also received an unexpected windfall when a Malvern lady named Christine van Gulik, who had never used the Hospice nor had any communication with its management team to anyone's knowledge, left more than £12.1 million in her will, to be equally split between 10 local charities, one of which was St Michael's.

With annual running costs back then coming in at around £1.8 million, it provided the Hospice with two thirds of its yearly income. It was also a reassuring reminder of just how highly St Michael's was now valued and regarded among the local community.

The Hospice Lottery made its first appearance in the year 2000, offering weekly prizes of £1,000, £200, £75 and £25, as well as £200 worth of £10 winners.

At that time, it was already costing £6,680 per day to keep the doors of St Michael's open, with 85% of that money needing to be raised locally.

Richard Shackelford, head of fundraising, spelled out the importance of the lottery in a letter to friends and volunteers in 2007.

"By the end of March 2007, our lottery members had raised a staggering £2 million for the Hospice. This is a fantastic amount.

"But if, by April 2007, every volunteer, support group member, trustee and staff member all managed to persuade just one friend to join and play every week in the coming year, we would either raise enough money to employ two full-time nurses, or pay for all the electricity and heating oil used at St Michael's."

Well over 6,000 people had signed up for the lottery at that time, and today, it has more than 7,500 members, and has raised a total of £5,275,000 for the Hospice.

Carl Attwood looks back on his time in the hot-seat as 'very, very happy'.

He says: "I see it as a massive privilege. There was never a time, even when we were going through the transition, that I thought to myself 'What am I doing here?'

"I'm a colourful and noisy type of character, and believed in having fun at meetings.

"But I could also be firm when the need arose, and remember many times when we were getting bogged down in administrative details and I had to remind everyone why we were here – for the patients!"

Ooh, matron!

Carl Attwood's successor in the chairman's seat was Sylvia Jones, a safe and knowledgeable pair of hands who had been involved with the Hospice since it was barely a year old.

Back then, Sylvia was deputy district nursing officer at the local health authority who was asked by her bosses to go into St Michael's and act as a part-time matron.

"Compared with the Hospice we see today, it was a very quiet place, with maybe only six or eight beds," she recalls.

"The previous matron had left, and they were looking for someone who could step in and handle some of her duties, as well as helping to smooth things over on the personnel side.

"Even in those early years, though, there was something special about the atmosphere. Music was playing, people were chatting, and although staff were working very hard, the mood was always light."

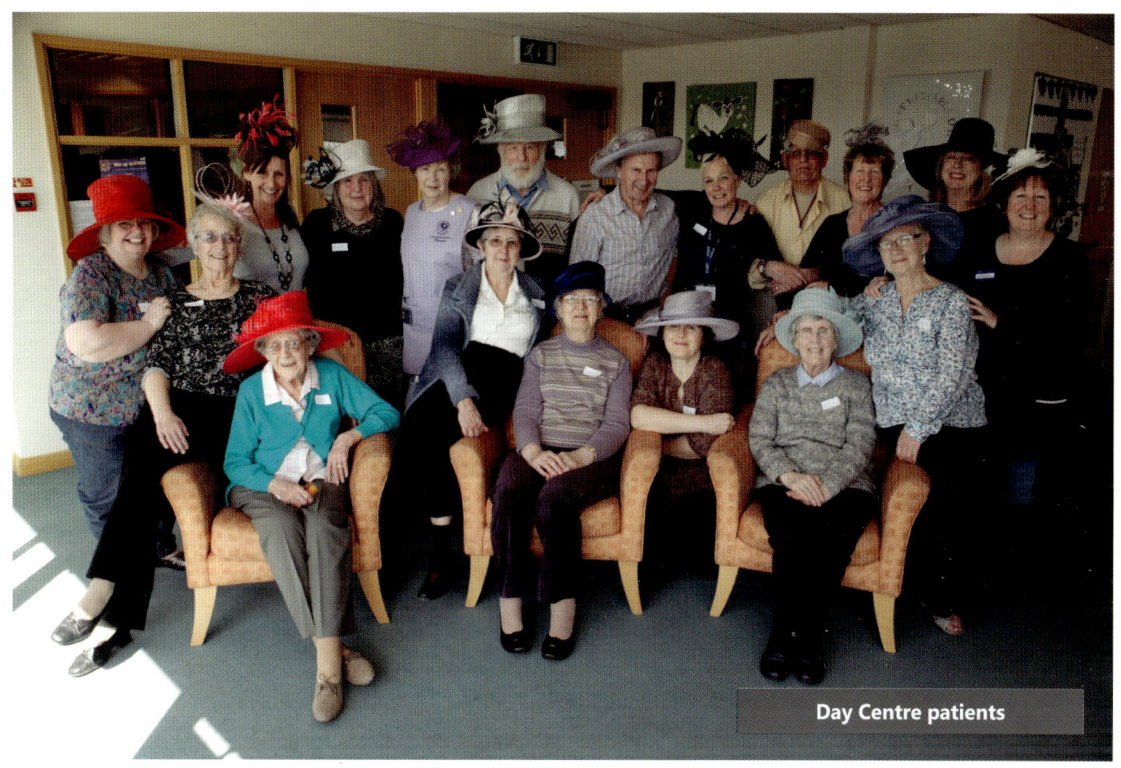

Day Centre patients

It wasn't long before Sylvia was invited to take up a seat on the Hospice board – something she was only too delighted to do. By then, she is happy to admit she was 'totally immersed' in hospice life, both as a professional adviser, and an enthusiastic volunteer.

"The Hospice has always been a place which puts patient care and sensitivity first, even though it had grown like topsy by this stage with fundraising activities like the lottery, and network of shops.

"The feedback we were getting from people who have been in the Hospice was so complimentary, and I was always proud to be associated with the team."

Walter Brooks was chief executive in its 20th anniversary year; by which time the public had gained a much better understanding of the role of hospices, and the high standards of care they provided.

"Those who set up the Hospice did not have that advantage," he wrote in the commemorative magazine.

"First, they had to persuade people that Herefordshire needed a Hospice at all; that it should be supported through voluntary subscription, and that they were the people to lead the initiative.

"And they had to do so without having any track record in this field to support their argument.

"The fact that they did so can only be described as heroic. They created the vision and they delivered it. They raised all the funds needed for the construction, plus 12 months of running costs. They acquired the land and they completed the building – all within five years of the first public meeting."

Two decades on, the Hospice was facing a similar type of challenge, though far less daunting than that faced by the founders.

Equipment for patient care had increased in both volume and size, and items like hoists, which were regarded as luxuries in those founding years, were now seen as essential.

Society's expectations had shifted too. Back in 1984, a luxurious room in tranquil surroundings, serviced by polite, experienced and sensitive staff ticked all the boxes.

By the year 2004, people also expected en suites in their rooms with toilet, washing and shower facilities as a bare minimum. Money clearly needed to be spent on the infrastructure.

Walter wrote: "As St Michael's reputation grew, so did its activity. Back in 1992 it employed about 50 people, most of whom were part-time nurses.

"In 2004, that figure was 96. In 1993, there were three charity shops, but by 2004 there were 13, with a 14th due to open.

"And so it went on . . . expenditure on Hospice services and their directly related costs amounted to more than £4,300 a day in 2004, and the total costs for running all activities was nearly £6,100 a day."

If an organisation such as St Michael's Hospice was to continue to maintain and, where possible improve its services, it needed a building fit for current standards in Palliative Care.

That meant not just catching up with the changes of the most recent past, but building in flexibility to cope with predicted advances in care over the next two decades.

There has never been any time to stand still at St Michael's.

Blooming marvellous

The custodians of St Michael's Hospice for the third decade in its history inherited a facility that had stood the test of time.

It was their job to re-invigorate that inheritance, build on the good work, and provide a facility that will continue to serve the people of Herefordshire and the surrounding areas well into the 21st century.

Looking back with respect, looking forward with excitement and enthusiasm, and marching on.

The Hospice celebrated its 25th anniversary in 2009. Much had changed during the passing of a quarter of a century, but the strength of the organisation still lay with the partnerships established with enthusiasts, volunteers and local companies.

With just 10 per cent of income coming from statutory bodies at that stage, the generosity of the local community was more important than ever in helping to maintain the high levels of care.

One of the highlights of the year was the Silver Jubilee Thanksgiving Service held in Hereford Cathedral, which saw an official Hospice Choir assembled for the first time.

Yes, long before the angelic Gareth Malone burst onto the reality TV scene, St Michael's was serving up its own version of The Choir, with a line-up comprising staff, volunteers and care beneficiaries.

Princess Alexandra, who had supported the cause from the very outset, made her third visit to the Hospice in July, going out of her way to speak to patients, staff and volunteers before being taken on a tour of the site to see some of the recent innovations, including

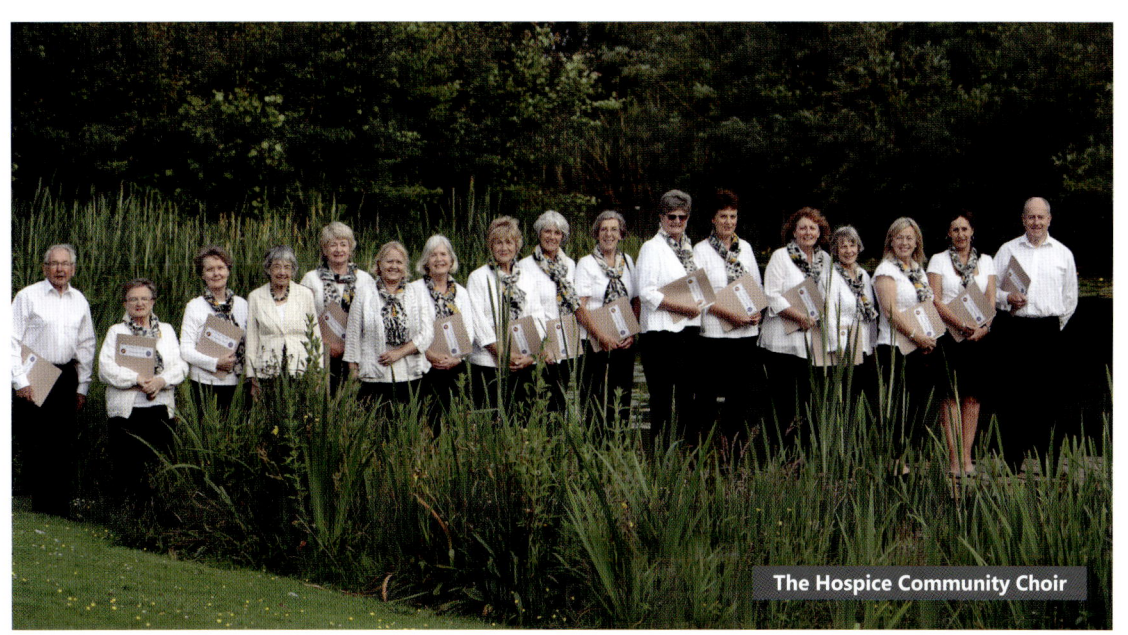

The Hospice Community Choir

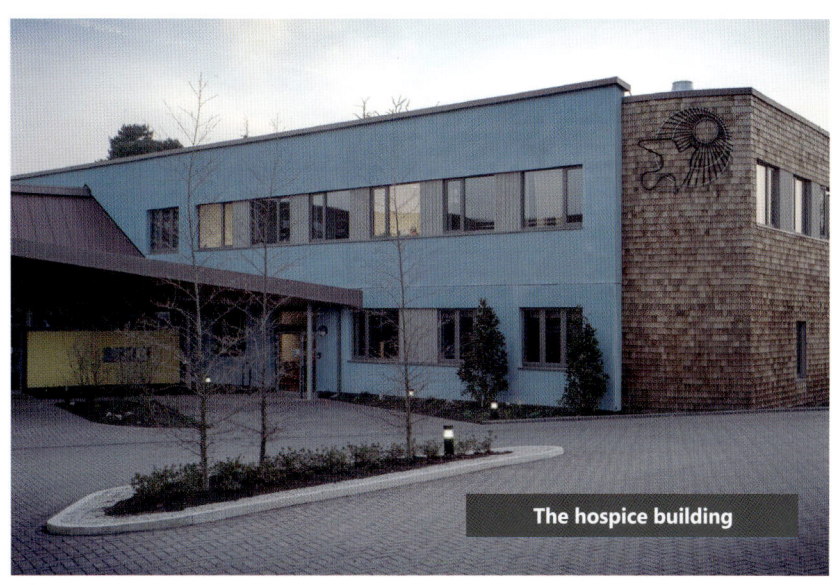

The hospice building

a new garden room and, 'the pod', an area designed specially for teenage visitors to the hospice.

From there, the Princess was taken to Lyde Arundel to see the magnificent celebratory flower festival, A Cornucopia of Silver, being held in the Hospice's honour, where she met more long-serving staff and volunteers.

Two flowers were produced specially for the celebratory year. One was a red rose called Precious Time, grown by C&K Jones of Cheshire and launched at Malvern Show by the BBC's Kate Bliss.

The other, Aster Novae Angliae St Michael's, was a September flowering Michaelmas daisy, created by Paul and Meriel Picton of Old Court Nurseries in Colwall.

The flower festival raised a blooming brilliant £72,000 for Hospice funds – but perhaps more importantly than that, it drew in many first-time volunteers who had not previously been involved, but who became loyal and long-standing supporters.

Sylvia Jones handed over the chairmanship to the current incumbent, Alister Walshe, heralding yet another exciting chapter of the Hospice's history . . . not to mention another big fundraising challenge.

The maverick estate agent

"One thing I do know about is bricks and mortar," says estate agency boss Alister Walshe, who runs Stooke Hill & Walshe in Hereford. "So, in many ways this was the perfect time for me to take over in the chair."

Alister first became involved with St Michael's at the turn of the century, while helping to care for one of his closest friends, who had been diagnosed with Motor Neurone Disease at the age of 33.

"He had a very aggressive form of the disease, and I would spend two or three hours with him, two or three times a week. We set about looking for somewhere which could provide the appropriate end of life care for him, and I knew of St Michael's."

Alister was soon immersed in Hospice affairs, and used his role as the chairman of the Hereford Round Table to help bring the garden to life.

He explains: "I made a pledge during my year as chairman that I would raise enough funds to do the garden, which was basically just a pile of rubble at the time.

"In conjunction with several businesses, we achieved the objective, raising money, and calling in favours." It turned into a true DIY SOS-style project.

Soon, Alister was on the board of trustees and was, by his own admission, 'well and truly hooked'.

"I'd become so passionate about what St Michael's was doing, and became chairman of the fundraising committee. I remember telling my wife that I'd probably only be attending four or five meetings a year, but before I knew it, I was finding myself there at some stage virtually every week. The place gets you like that."

When Sylvia Jones handed the chairmanship of the St Michael's board over to Alister exciting redevelopment plans were already on the drawing board.

"Just before I became a trustee there had been talk of a redevelopment to provide a

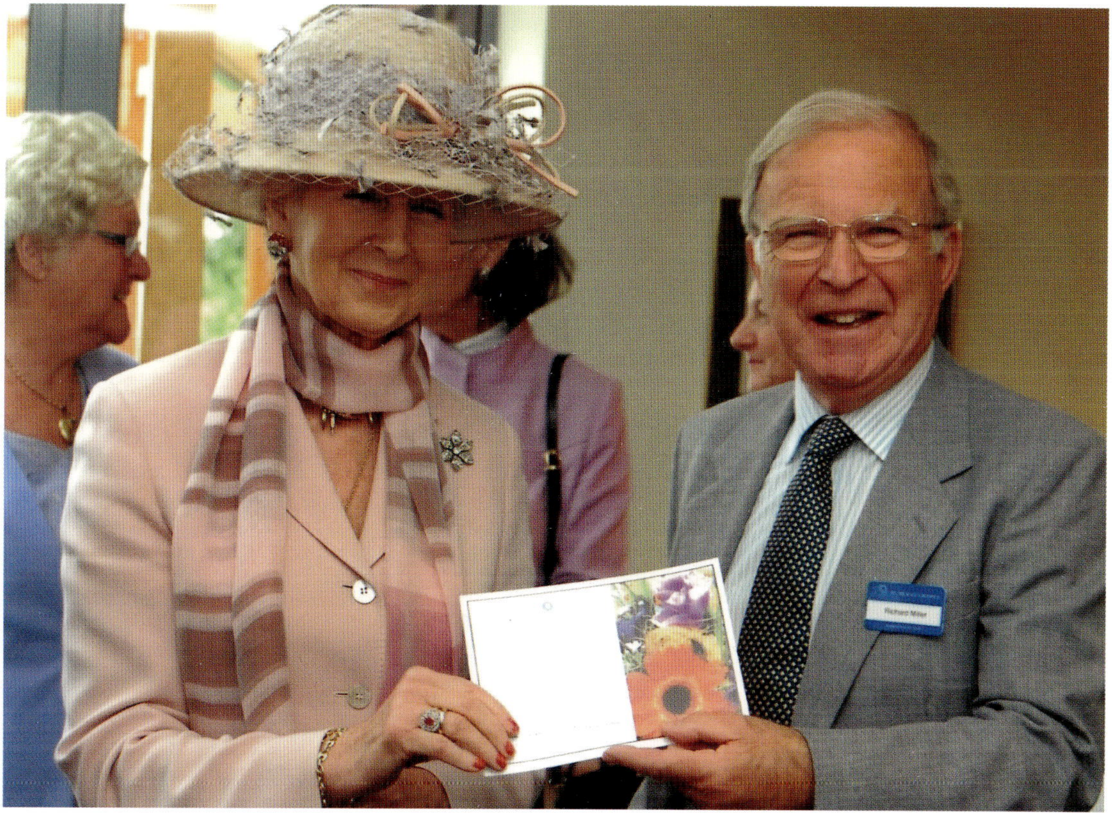

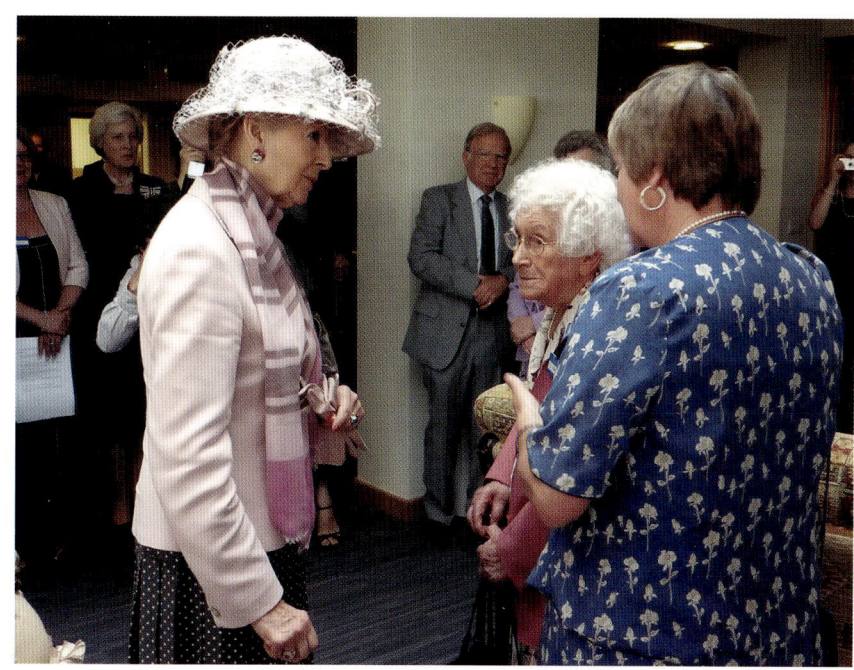

Princess Alexandra's visit to celebrate the Hospice's 25th Anniversary in 2009

new in-patient wing, but for one reason or another it had been put on the back-burner," Alister says.

"I made it my mission, during my time as chairman, to make it happen, knowing the depth of support which existed among the wonderful people of Herefordshire. I think I took a fairly maverick approach to it all.

"Through my estate agency profession, I know all about building properties – how much they cost, the challenges, pitfalls and implications. So this was a perfect time for me to put my skills and experience to good use."

In addition to overseeing the plans for the expansion, Alister also negotiated the purchase of three new houses in the convent grounds.

The initial idea was to keep them for a few years to provide support facilities for the Hospice during building work, then sell them off at a profit to help pay for the building costs.

But healthy fundraising activities – spearheaded by the increasingly successful network of shops – mean St Michael's now looks likely to be able to hold onto them permanently.

"The phenomenal fundraising is giving us so much more flexibility," Alister says. "We can use the three houses, for example, to provide accommodation for families travelling from a long way away, or for relatives who want to spend some time off-site

Alister says he has worked hard to create a blend of youthful enthusiasm, and sagely experience on the current St Michael's board.

"You should never overlook the importance of experience and maturity, but you also need younger people who have inside knowledge on what is happening in the business world at the moment.

"I feel very lucky to have support from such a hard-working and loyal group of trustees, who share my complete passion for St Michael's."

One of Alister's remaining big ambitions during his chairmanship is to see Hospice teams being able to reach out to patients at an even earlier stage in their end-of-life journey.

"St Michael's is very much part of the community, and exists thanks to their amazing efforts. So the more we can do for the people, the more they will hopefully see that the support they have given to us over the years has been justified, and so worthwhile."

Renovation, and redevelopment

As the 30th anniversary year approached, St Michael's had become something of a victim of its own success, and its widening reputation for excellence.

Demand was outstripping the ability to supply, so in 2013 the Board of Trustees launched a Redevelopment Appeal to build a much needed state-of-the-art expansion, adjoining the original Hospice building at Bartestree.

Once again, supporters rose magnificently to the challenge of raising the necessary funds, greatly helped by several incredibly generous legacies and charitable donations, and co-ordinated by the Hospice's head of fundraising, Ruth Denison, who is constantly driving forward with creative new ideas.

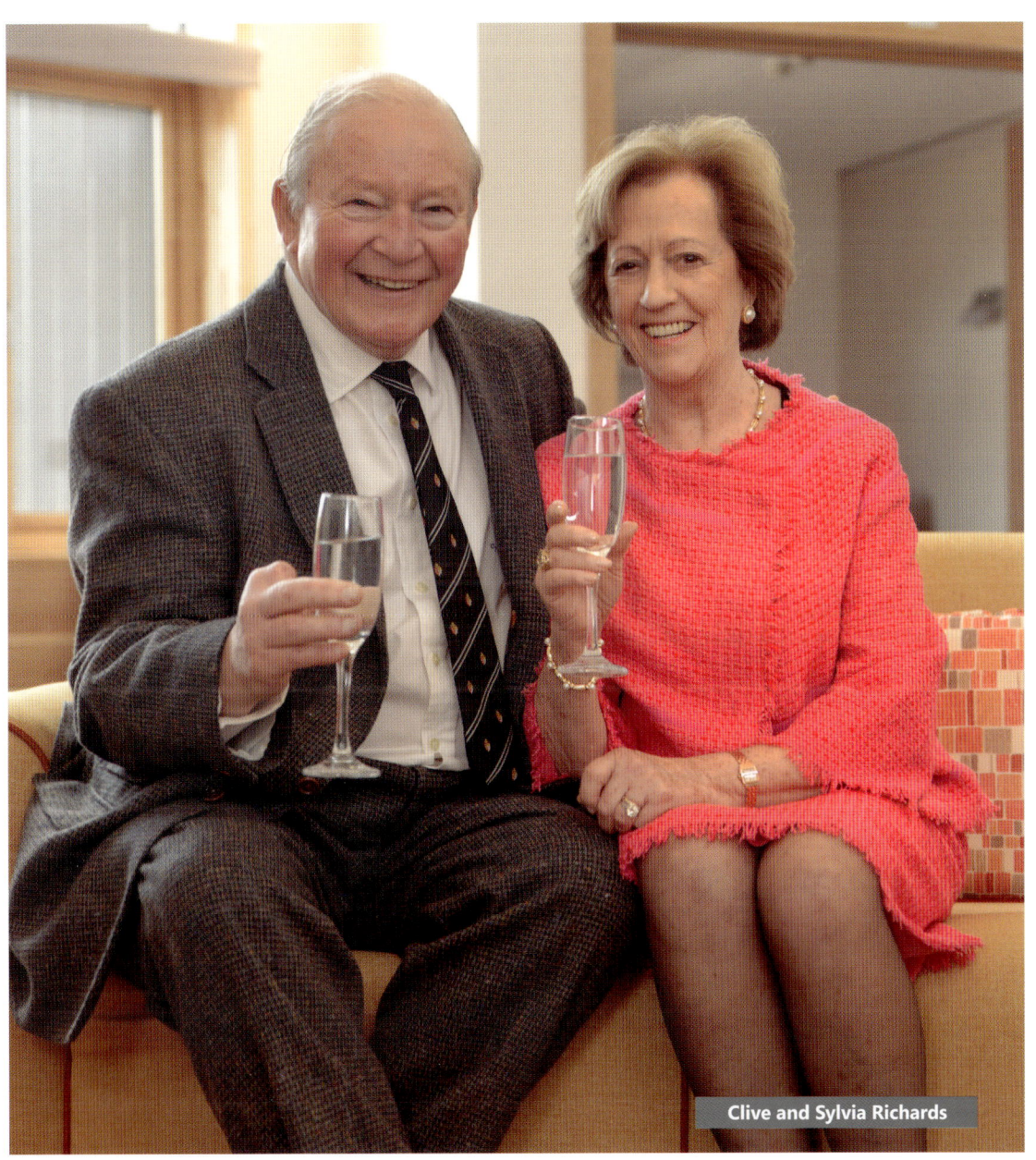

Clive and Sylvia Richards

To create the right kind of therapeutic environment, the design team gave just as much thought to the surrounding landscape as they did to the building.

With views looking across beautiful rolling Herefordshire countryside, the wildlife-friendly gardens at the new Hospice were designed to provide a restful and peaceful environment for patients, their friends, and family.

Rainwater-collecting channels now twist and fall through a variety of plants and trees which have been planted in the grounds to reflect the colour and texture of the new building.

Water features, which surround the patient clusters, are fed by the rain that falls on the cedar shingle roof – all part of a landscape designed to provide a sensory environment for all who spend time at St Michael's.

The Clive and Sylvia Richards Charity generously donated £1 million towards the project. Clive Richards, who describes himself as a 'serial entrepreneur', established the charity, with his wife Sylvia, in 1986.

The charity's focus is to support Education, Healthcare, Heritage, Arts, Religious Institutions and Overseas Education and Religious Institutions.

In recognition of their generosity, Clive and Sylvia were invited to officially open the new in-patient unit at the end of March 2015.

Mr Richards said: 'St Michael's is built on the generosity of tens of thousands of people who have supported their Hospice over the last 30 years.

"I knew that raising the funds for the redevelopment was going to be a massive challenge and I wanted to encourage people to get behind the project. I also wanted to show people just how inspirational their dedication to St Michael's Hospice has been

for me personally."

Built to the highest engineering standards, every aspect of the highly insulated, timber-framed building was considered to ensure St Michael's continues to meet the needs of the local community for generations to come.

Chief executive during this time was Nicky West, who spent nearly a decade at the helm before stepping down in September 2015.

One of her biggest contributions was the development and implementation of a 'Hospice at Home' service which brought together different healthcare providers to help people to continue living well at home for as long as possible.

Nicky recognised that the old Hospice building, first opened in 1984, was in need of a major redevelopment. And, having kept a safe and steady hand on the tiller during the £11.3 million redevelopment appeal, and with the completion of the first phase of the new inpatient unit and refurbishment of the old building well underway, she felt the time was right to move on.

She says: "I am incredibly privileged to have worked with a team of truly wonderful people. I know how important St Michael's Hospice is to the local community and my inspiration has always come from the thousands of people who have supported their Hospice in so many inspiring ways.

"I would like to thank everyone who has helped make St Michael's Hospice a place of light and love and I know that with so many truly exceptional people involved it will continue to care for local families for generations to come."

Colleagues praised Nicky's vision and motivational leadership, which they said had helped shape a hospice that offers so much more than just nursing and medicine.

Her instinctive understanding of what was

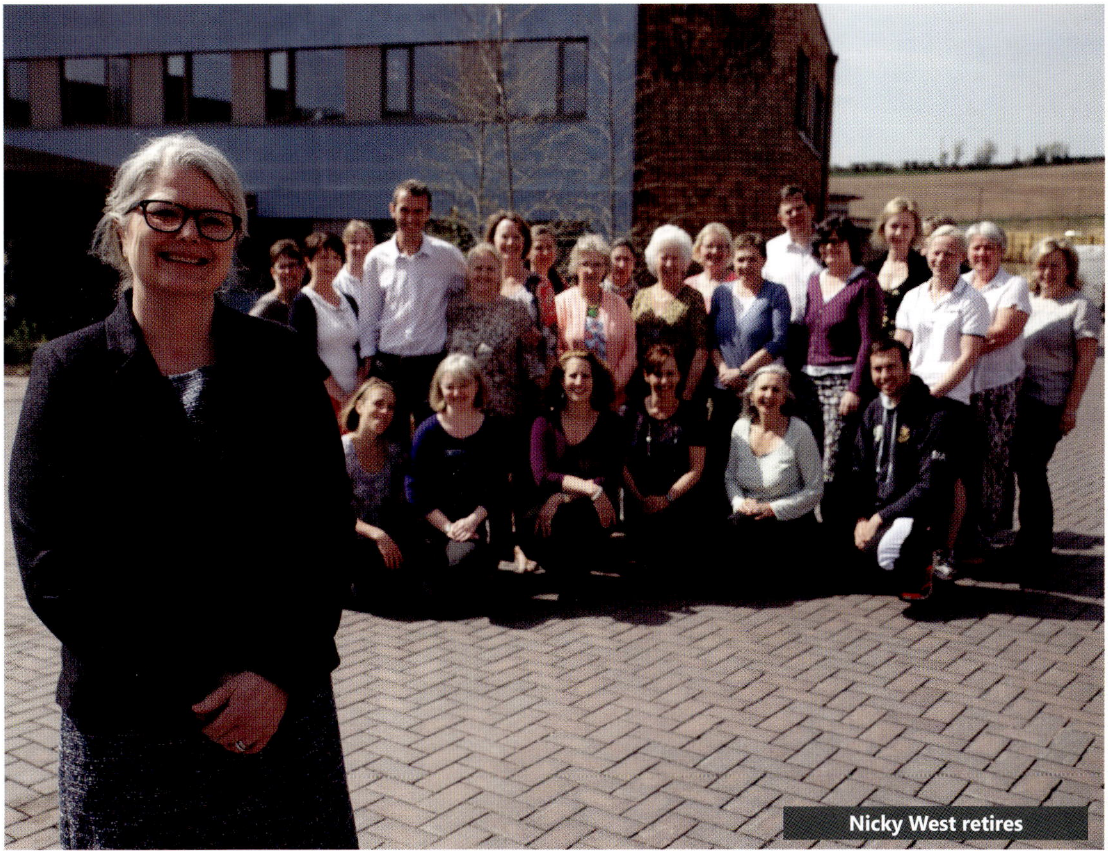

Nicky West retires

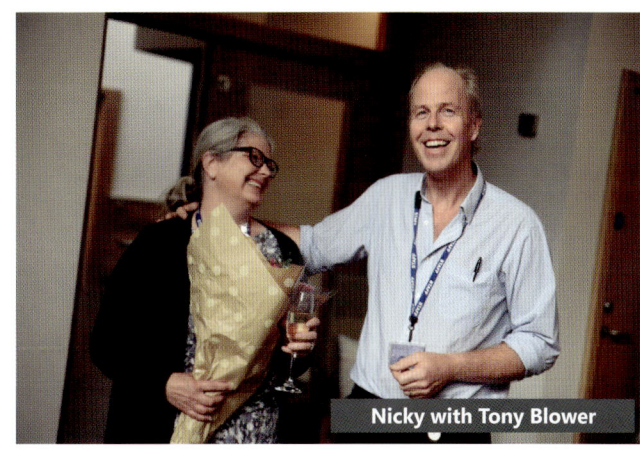

Nicky with Tony Blower

needed, and the tenacity to get stuck into the nitty-gritty to make things happen, are the enduring memory for her numerous St Michael's friends.

When a plan comes together...

Health Care Assistant Debbie Emmett first began working at St Michael's over 15 years ago.

Comparing the difference between 'then' and 'now', she says: "When I began working at St Michael's 15 years ago, the Hospice was much quieter.

"Today there is a much greater need for all our services, and we are caring for more people in many different ways. Patients can now visit us for symptom control and then return home, and many more patients will soon be able to use our in-reach services, enabling people to live in their own homes for as long as possible."

One of the key design features of the new building is private bedrooms with en-suite bathrooms. Debbie believes this feature is vital to help care for people with the dignity they deserve.

"I can't emphasise enough the difference the extra space and facilities will make to the quality of people's lives during their stay at the Hospice."

The bespoke building was one of the most challenging and ultimately rewarding projects for Architype, the Herefordshire-based architects who have designed the build.

After listening to Hospice staff, patients, families and friends, Architype designed a building that engages the senses and provides a truly astonishing therapeutic environment. The technology used will reduce running costs, making the building affordable to run.

Architect Paul Neep said: "St Michael's Hospice has touched the lives of so many people in Herefordshire; it has been a privilege to help create this beautiful new facility that will enable the Hospice to provide a quiet, comfortable and relaxing environment whilst avoiding clinical uniformity."

Just as much thought has been given to the external environment.

Landscape architects have created streams for rainwater to run through and rills to act as therapeutic water features, offering sound and visual animation to help soothe and calm.

Carefully planted flowers, shrubs and hedgerows help to link the building into its location in the stunning Herefordshire countryside.

The second stage of the redevelopment project – the refurbishment of the existing building – is now nearing completion.

The end result is a hospice which is truly fit for the 21st century, providing all the space needed to care for and support people living with a life-limiting illness, whether in their own homes or as inpatients.

Pat Rawson, who started volunteering at St Michael's in the mid 1980s, says: "When I walked into the new building for the first time, I knew instantly it was a place where the tradition of caring for the community will continue to be second to none."

But the St Michael's mission for the future – to continue to revolutionise palliative care and support more local families with a broadened range of services – was never

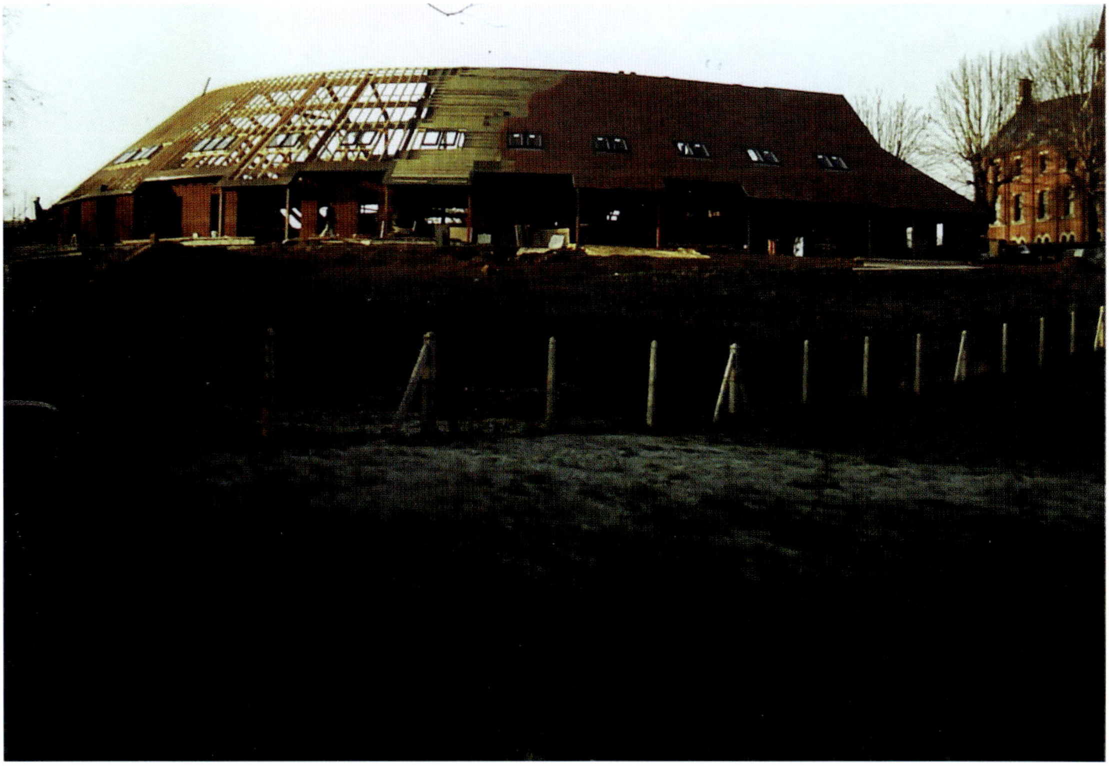

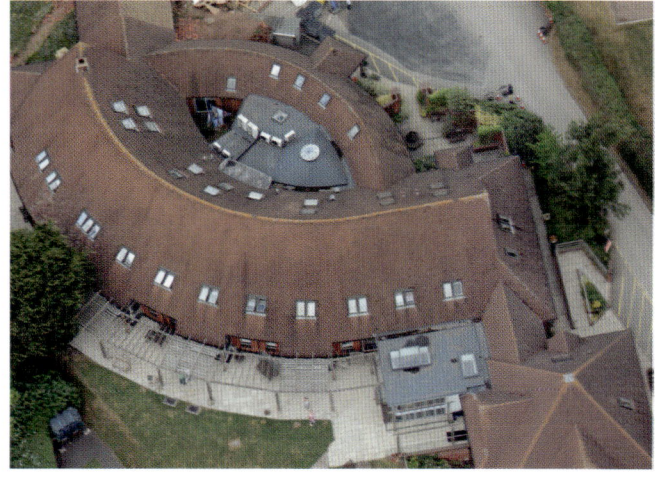

A modern hospice

going to be cheap.

It costs more than £13,000 a day to continue to provide free of charge care to patients at St Michael's Hospice. If you do the maths, you'll realise that this comes in at more than £4.7 million a year.

Almost 90 per cent of this comes in from the community, in the form of legacies, events, plus the network of shops, and the weekly lottery.

The success of the St Michael's charity shop network has been nothing short of phenomenal. There are now 17 stores, based in Hereford and a host of surrounding towns and villages including Tenbury Wells, Kington, Ross-on-Wye, Ledbury, Presteigne, Malvern, Hay-on-Wye, Leominster and Bromyard.

In August 2015, the shop network won the 'Most Profitable Charity Retail Operation' award in the prestigious National Charity Retail Awards, having contributed more than £1.2 million in just 12 months.

Mary Brown, Volunteer Manager at Eign Gate Shop in Hereford, said: "Volunteering for St Michael's feels like having a second family. It has given me the chance to give something back to the Hospice movement in return for the unparalleled care given to my partner.

"It's the best therapy I could have had. I wouldn't give it up for all the tea in China. Many of the people I work with have experienced similar situations and winning this award as a team is very special."

And Nicola Wood, head of retail at St Michael's, added: "I'm very proud of everyone involved. Over the last 15 years, St Michael's has needed to provide more and more services to local families. Because of the volunteers, staff and the thousands of people who have donated quality goods, the Hospice can provide more families with the care they need."

A large proportion of the goods sold through the shops benefits from Gift Aid, a Government scheme which enables charities to reclaim 25p of every £1 donated by tax-paying individuals. The scheme also allows charities to reclaim 25% of the sale price of donated goods sold in charity shops.

For St Michael's Hospice, this amounts to a whopping £100,000 that could potentially be recovered from the Inland Revenue if all its donors were registered for Gift Aid – that's why volunteers are always so keen to urge supporters to fill in the magic form every time they bring goods in for sale.

It's OK to laugh, and OK to cry…

Ask the average person in the street about the role of a hospice, and they will speak fondly of the support it provides for people with cancer, and other terminal illness.

But in many ways, that is just the tip of the iceberg; in the modern-day world, facilities like St Michael's provide much, much more than that.

The Family Support Team has an increasingly pivotal role, reaching out to children, parents, carers and relatives of those with life-limiting illnesses, ensuring they get the help they need to plot a path through whatever the future may hold . . . and at the

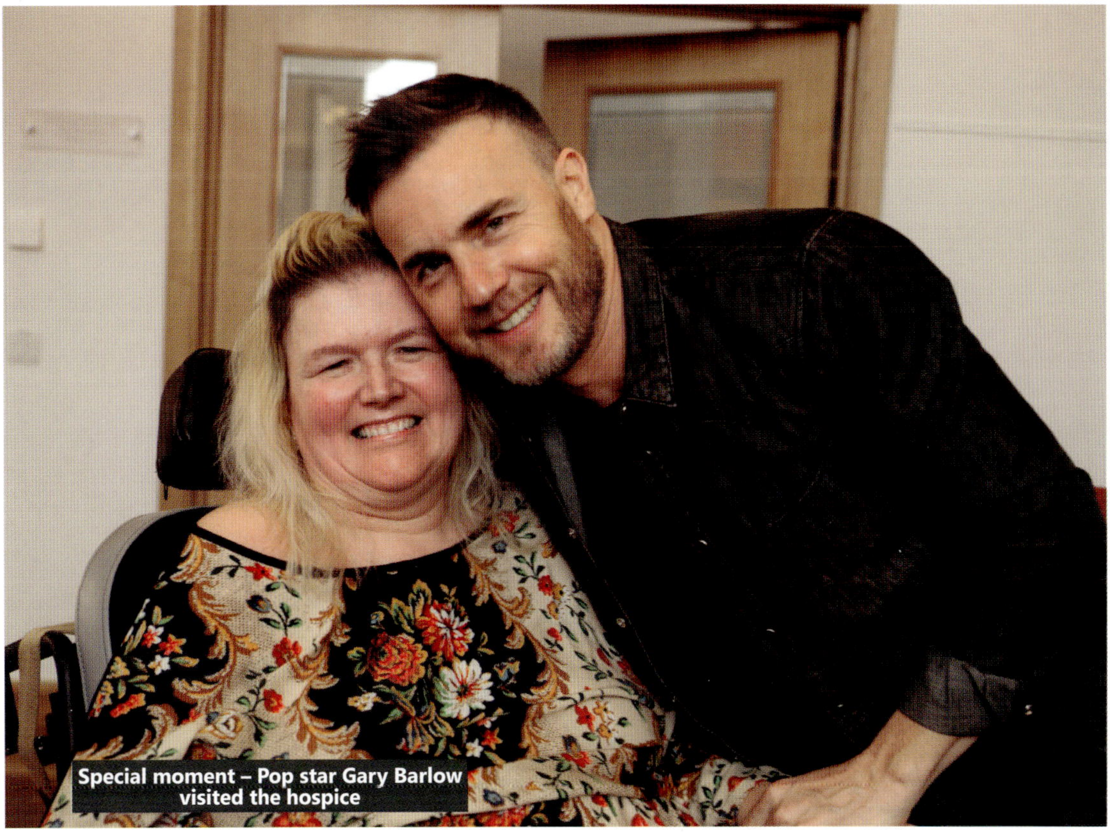

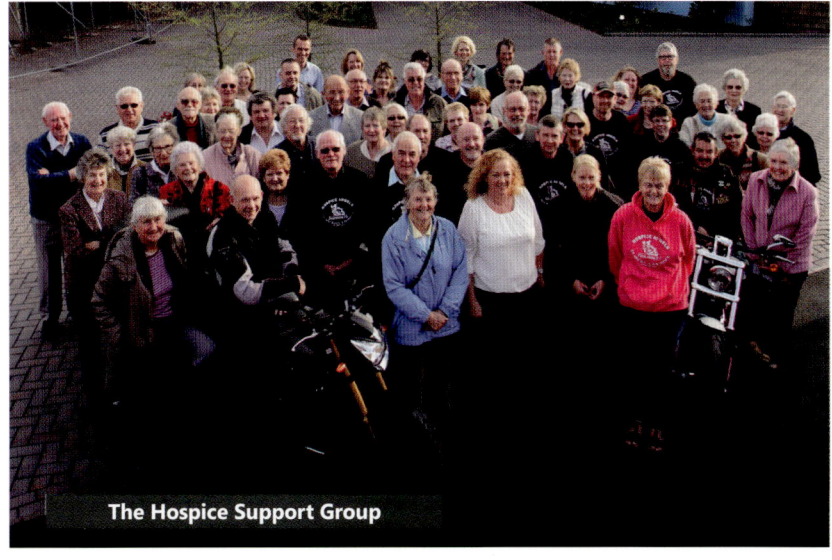

Special moment – Pop star Gary Barlow
visited the hospice

The Hospice Support Group

earliest possible opportunity.

Sometimes, that might simply be a shoulder to cry on, a kind word, a chaplaincy service, or the creation of an environment in which people feel safe enough to express their bottled-up feelings.

But it can also be far more strategic than that – working over prolonged periods with families and outside agencies to plan for, and to tackle, the sometimes seismic changes to people's lives.

The Family Support Team at St Michael's is not simply staffed by nurses and medical staff; it includes experts with social work backgrounds too.

Between them, they have developed a wide-ranging menu of social care, emotional support, and both pre and post-bereavement help to people of all ages, recognising the different type of assistance often required by parents, couples, children, or families as a whole.

When what has been seen as a 'normal' family life is changing, people need to feel able to ask questions, receive honest answers . . . and most importantly of all, be reassured that they are not alone.

It's OK to laugh at St Michael's Hospice. And it's OK to cry too. Laughter is often one of the most effective forms of therapy, and dark humour is regularly used to diffuse the most awful situations.

But the ethos at St Michael's is that, whatever emotion people feel the urge to express, it is absolutely fine. No-one is judged.

That's because the team recognise the tremendous sense of freedom and empowerment which comes from feeling completely secure, and solidly supported.

The Family Support Team knows it can't make the pain of what has happened – or

is going to happen – go away. But it can be alongside those affected, and can help to foster the belief that things will become easier.

Sara Higginson was one of the pioneers of this bereavement support service, working at St Michael's for more than 20 years before her retirement in 2013.

She, and the team she helped to build, reassure friends and family members that, in one way or another, they will make it through, and there will be someone beside them every step of the way.

"When I arrived, I was particularly keen to put a greater focus on the needs of young children," she says.

"They often end up being called upon to do things they would not normally be expected to do at such a young age. I'm not saying that it is common for patients to be in their 30s rather than their 60s or 70s, but it happens more often than you might think.

"And if a parent is ill – particularly when they are younger – you have to enable the children to feel they can ask mummy and daddy, or their grandparents, what will happen to them.

"Children need to know what it is going to mean for them. Who will they live with, for example? But there is still a stigma surrounding 'The Big C', and people don't find it easy to talk about it.

"Without having these sorts of conversations, though, children can often have a very confused understanding of what was happening in their lives – and parents, and other adult carers like aunts, uncles and grandparents, don't really know what to say to them.

"We have spent a lot of time working with staff at St Michael's, giving them the confidence to talk to children – as well as

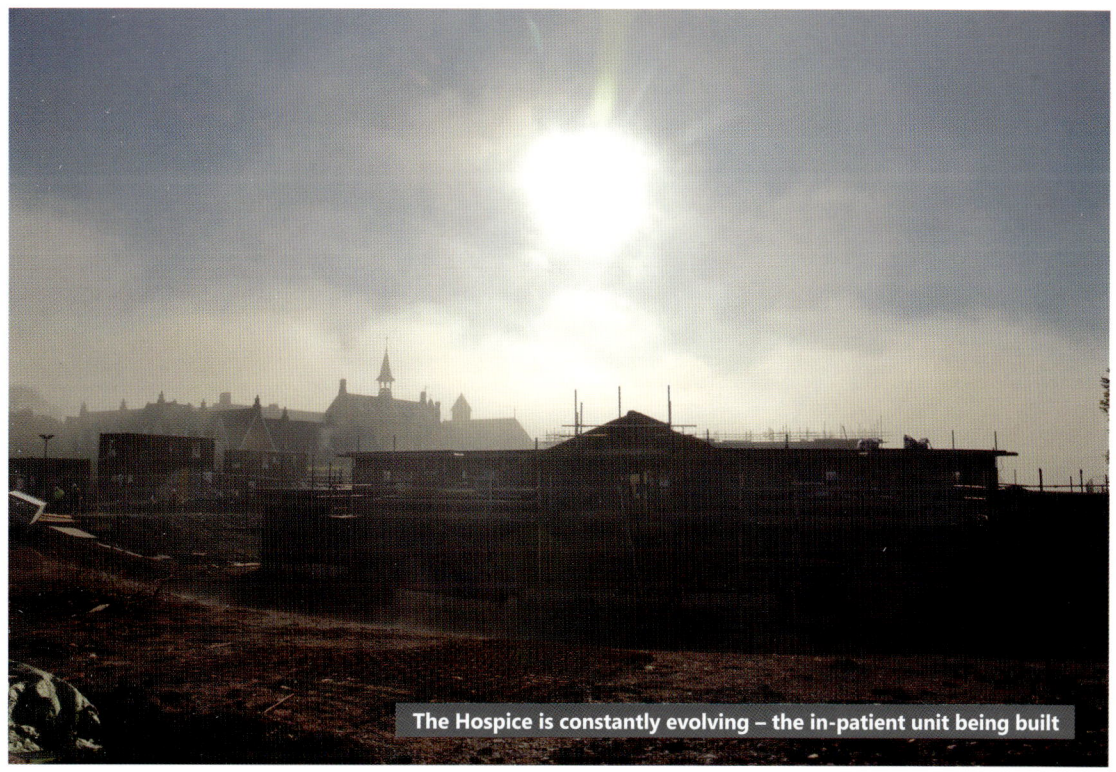

The Hospice is constantly evolving – the in-patient unit being built

explaining to their parents why it is important to have these difficult conversations with their own children, while they can.

"When I first arrived here, I was very concerned that nobody was asking children what they knew, what they understood, or explained to them what was happening with the doctors and nurses they saw coming and going. That has changed dramatically over the years – particularly during Nicky West's time as chief executive. She understood our vision, and gave us tremendous support."

Saturday Club is one of the many innovations. There is a monthly club for five–11 year-olds, as well as regular evening support groups for those aged 12-16, and 17-25.

They are divided, where possible, into sessions for those whose loved ones are still ill, and those who have been through a bereavement.

One-to-one support is offered to under-fives, primary school-aged children, teens and young adults, and there is a busy programme of activity days, trips and workshops, as well as home visits in many circumstances.

But it doesn't end there. The St Michael's team also provides support and training for teachers and other education professionals, and works closely with many support agencies.

This could simply involve informing schools, colleges or workplaces when someone is a young carer, and ensuring staff are supporting them in an appropriate way.

Sara, who is still involved with St Michael's through voluntary work at its twinned hospice, Muheza in Tanzania, adds: "One of the most moving things during my time was a letter which I received from one family member.

"It spoke of how much they recognised and appreciated the work we were doing with children, and the difference we had made. 'I couldn't do it, but I admire what a brilliant job your team are doing', it said. That meant such a lot.

"We also have people who tell us 'We wish we had known about this place earlier'. A hospice should not be seen simply as a place where people only come to spend their final few days, which is why we now seek to reach out to people at a much earlier stage of their illness.

"That is probably one of the biggest changes over the past decade, and it is very important to the wider family.

"If we can develop a relationship with them, and their children, at an earlier point, they become used to the Hospice and its staff, and experience tells us that, as a result, they find things far less traumatic."

Educating, and innovating

The hospice movement has always held a strong commitment to education and training: Dame Cicely Saunders, the nurse, social worker, physician and writer who pioneered the movement in the 1960s, believed education and research should form one of the cornerstones of care provision.

Her view is shared by Jean Fisher, the former plastic surgery and burns specialist who has been an integral part of the St Michael's team virtually since the start.

Jean arrived at St Michael's via something of a circuitous route. Originally from Hampshire, she had been working in Essex, and was keen to broaden her healthcare experience.

"We were caring for dying and terminally ill patients as part of my job, but I have to say we were not very good at it," she says.

"I'd been to Hereford only once – to a friend's wedding – but remembered what a beautiful part of the country it was. So, when the opportunity came up to become ward sister at St Michael's, I was delighted."

Jean took up the role in September 1984, expecting to spend a couple of years enhancing her knowledge of palliative care before returning to the NHS to share her new-found experience.

That was more than 30 years ago . . . and she's still immersed in life at St Michael's!

"After seven years as ward sister, I was given the chance to become clinical teacher, and to officially launch a new education service. When we started, back in 1990, it was just me.

"The team is still a small one – I'm supported by one person working three days a week, and a full time administrator – but we have made huge strides forward."

The St Michael's education service, under Jean's stewardship, became the first in the land to offer university-accredited training in Palliative and End of Life Care for people with a non-cancer diagnosis.

It is, in Jean's words, an 'any time, any place, anywhere' service, delivering training either in dedicated classrooms at St Michael's,

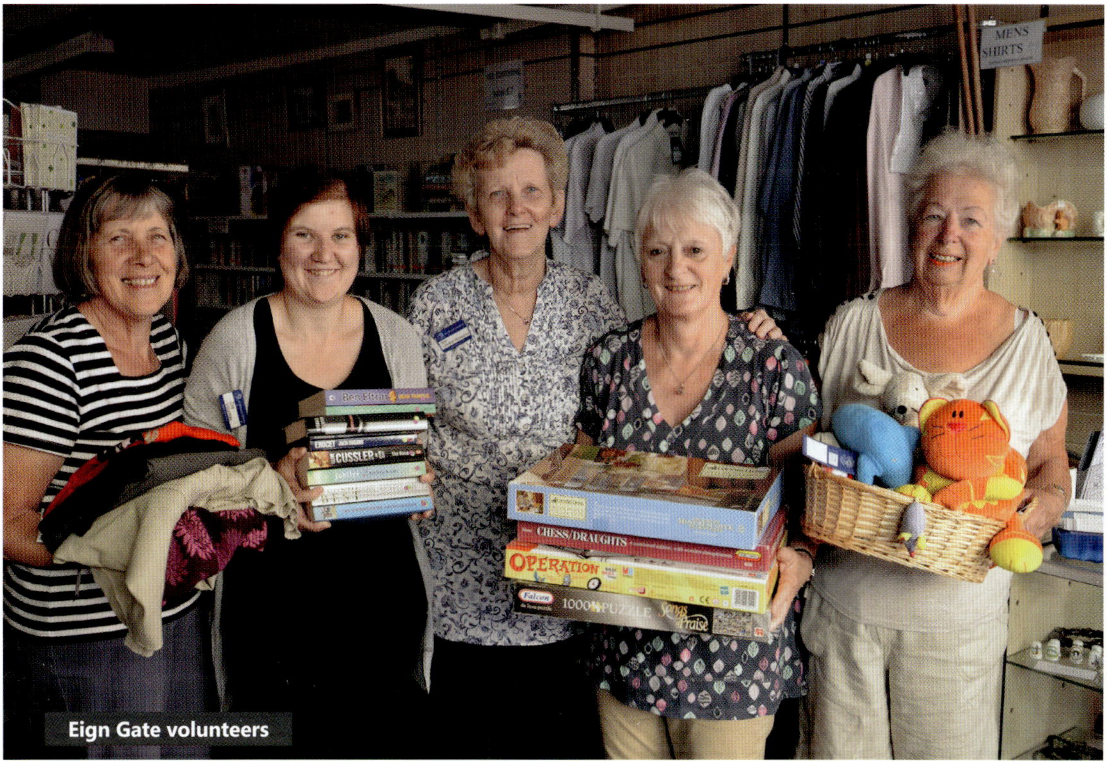

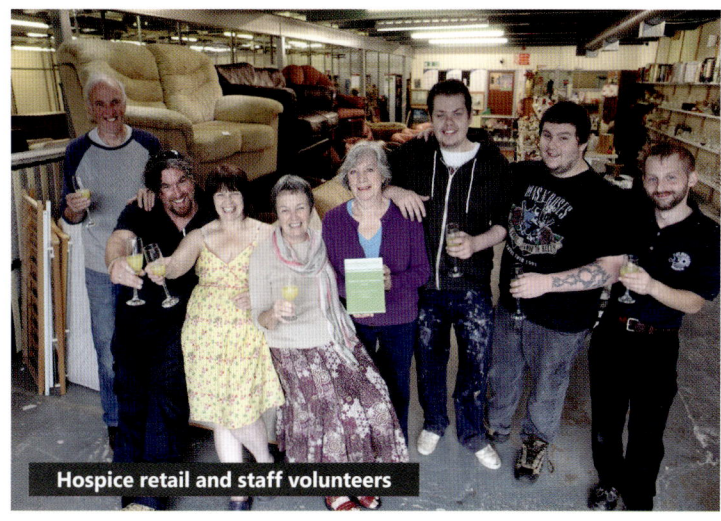

Eign Gate volunteers

Hospice retail and staff volunteers

or remotely on a client's premises.

She explains: "The objective of our education programmes is to widen the general awareness of what hospices, do, and to enhance the knowledge of professionals about palliative care, and the ways in which they can improve the way they care for end of life patients.

"Our core message has remained unchanged over the years – we are imparting knowledge, and trying to change people's attitudes.

"But the size of the operation here at St Michael's has grown too. Back in the early years, people were only referring patients to us at the very end of their lives, and we were hardly ever discharging people. They tended to only have weeks, or a maximum of one or two months, left.

"Now, more people are referred to us much earlier, meaning we are often in a position to support them for a period, and then discharge them back home.

"I'd like to think that the education programmes that we have been running are in some part responsible for a better understanding among the medical profession about how St Michael's can help."

As the needs of our community change, so the Hospice has always sought to change to meet those needs. The training and preparation of new and existing volunteer groups have helped to develop and offer new services such as the Hospice Neighbours service.

The St Michael's team believes it is vital to share knowledge, experience and understanding with other professionals, and to learn from them in turn. Spreading best practice.

Thanks to the work done by Jean and her team, the education support for professional staff is now embraced by nurses, doctors and many other professional disciplines, and offered both within the Hospice and off-site at GP practices, hospitals, care homes and agencies.

With the ever-increasing strains being placed on the National Health Service in the UK, and the ageing British population, the Hospice is acutely aware of how important its education modules can also be for families and informal carers.

It considers supporting individuals who find themselves in the position of carer as crucially important; that's why it has developed several dedicated support groups – and why those houses which the Hospice now owns could turn out to be a precious long-term investment.

Within the wider community, St Michael's also works with various organisations including schools and colleges, while outreach training is now being delivered in nursing homes, doctor's surgeries, community hospitals and other caregiving organisations . . . all tailored to the needs of the team, either in single or multiple sessions.

"Sharing what we learn can only help others, whether they are professional or lay carers, thereby improving the care and support of all in our community, today and in the future," Jean Fisher says.

Richard Miller adds: "I am passionate about the Hospice sharing its expertise with the wider caring community; Jean is too modest to admit it, but she and her team have established an Education Department of such excellence that it has done much to enhance St Michael's reputation both in the UK and internationally."

Which brings us back to the hospice in Muheza, Tanzania – an amazing facility, founded by an incredible lady.

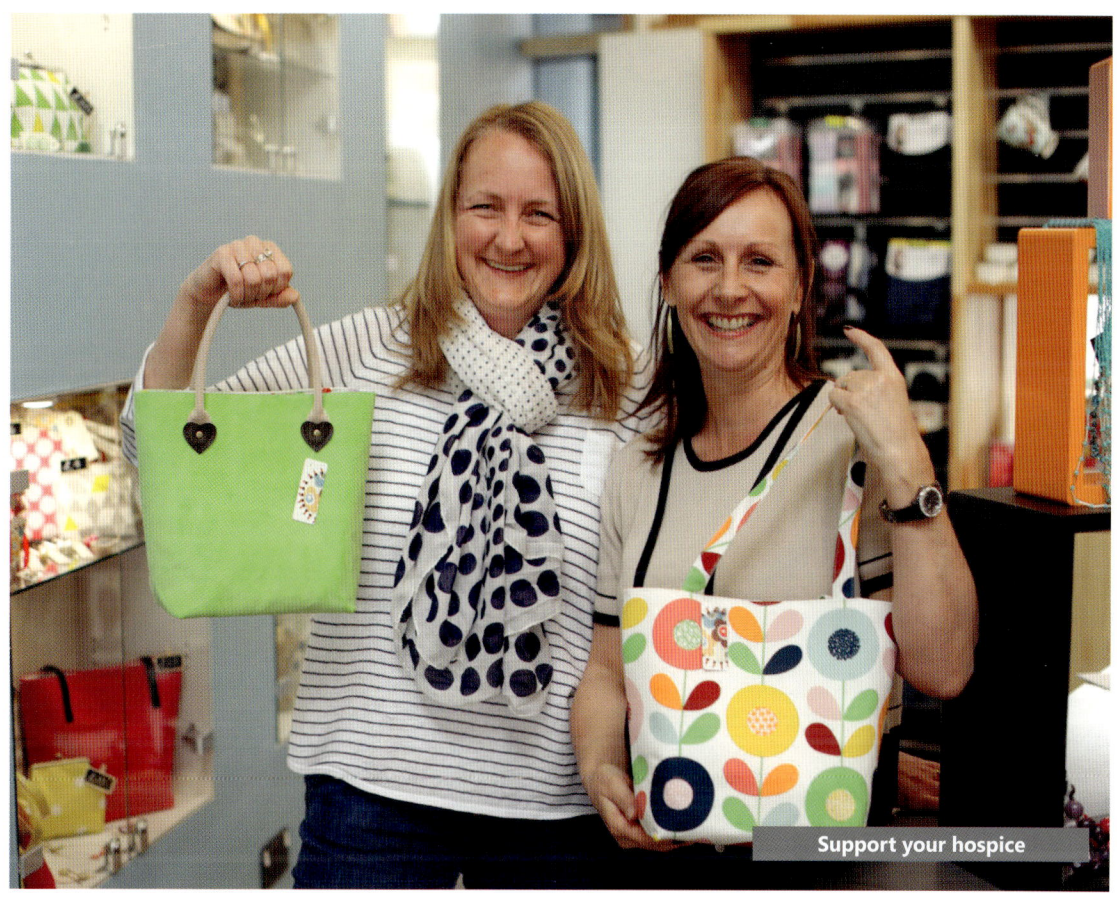

Support your hospice

In 2001, palliative care physician doctors Karilyn and Richard Collins retired from practice in the Leominster and Bodenham areas of Herefordshire to take up jobs at Teule hospital in Muheza.

Richard became medical superintendent and senior physician, and Karilyn could see a huge need for palliative care within the hospital and the community. That is how, and why, Muheza Hospice Care was born.

The couple returned to the UK in 2006, but have continued to visit the hospital frequently and take an interest in both the hospital and the hospice ever since. Karilyn has received the MBE for her services to palliative care, and a strong bond continues to exist between staff at St Michael's and their twinned centre in Tanzania.

The unpaid heroes

One common thread links every chapter of this amazing history; the contribution made by unpaid members of the local community to the St Michael's cause.

None of it would be possible without the continued backing of an army of volunteers who help in every aspect of Hospice life.

One man who knows this better than most is Stephen Rabbitts. The phrase 'been there, done that' was practically invented for Stephen, because there are few tasks that he hasn't thrown himself into during the 30-plus years he has been involved with St Michael's.

Stephen has been Head of Support Services for more than a decade now, having begun as one of the army of hard-working volunteers who helped to get the Hospice off the ground.

"My experience as a volunteer was incredibly challenging but so rewarding," he says. Over the past 30 years there has been a real increase in the number of volunteers we need to make St Michael's work every day.

"All our volunteers come with such a diversity of skills, experience and personality that they enhance the standard of care we are able to offer.

"I am constantly impressed when young volunteers join us as well. We have quite an age range in the 800-odd army that make up our corps of volunteers.

On his role as Head of Support Services, Stephen says: "It is extremely important to us here at the Hospice that the first impression created is a favourable one. Patients and their visitors often comment on our homely atmosphere, which is thanks to the efforts and high standards of our domestic team."

The increasing number of relatives who are now staying at the Hospice has placed a greater emphasis on the support network of domestic and kitchen staff.

Stephen says: "Support Services consists of a combination of paid staff and many volunteers who bring a wide range of skills to the Hospice. Our domestic staff do an excellent job ensuring that St Michael's gives that welcoming and homely atmosphere, which is essential when patients and relatives are apprehensive about coming into the hospice environment for the first time.

"Patients are our number one priority, and our catering team continues to provide healthy and delicious meals by consulting with patients and their relatives to ensure all their nutritional needs, special diets and tastes are catered for.

"They also continue to prepare meals for relatives, volunteers and staff, and support special events such as birthdays or anniversaries."

Stephen adds: "If you were to ask how the Hospice would operate without the help and support from our volunteers, the answer would be 'with great difficulty'.

"The volunteers work in the Hospice as receptionists, home makers, drivers, gardeners, nurses – in fact, in all areas of the organisation, a volunteer can be found working alongside paid members of staff.

"It creates a unique environment. In a typical year, we receive well over 20,000 hours of support from our volunteers. Imagine how much that would cost to employ paid staff. The value of our volunteers is quite simply immeasurable."

As is the contribution which St Michael's Hospice has made to the lives of so many people since first opening its doors, all those years ago.

———————————————

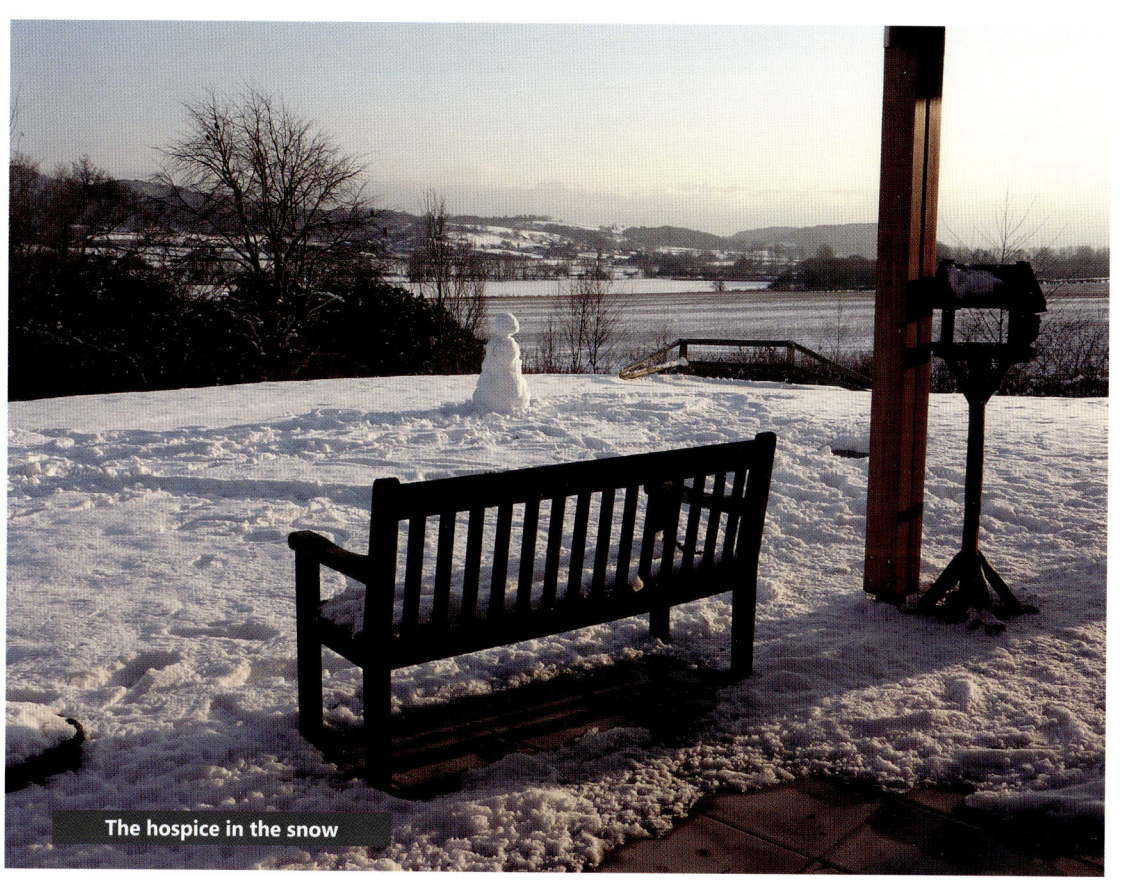

The hospice in the snow

Life and Hope at St Michael's Hospice

Olwyn Barnett, 79 Formerly Kinsham

By Debbie McMenemy, daughter

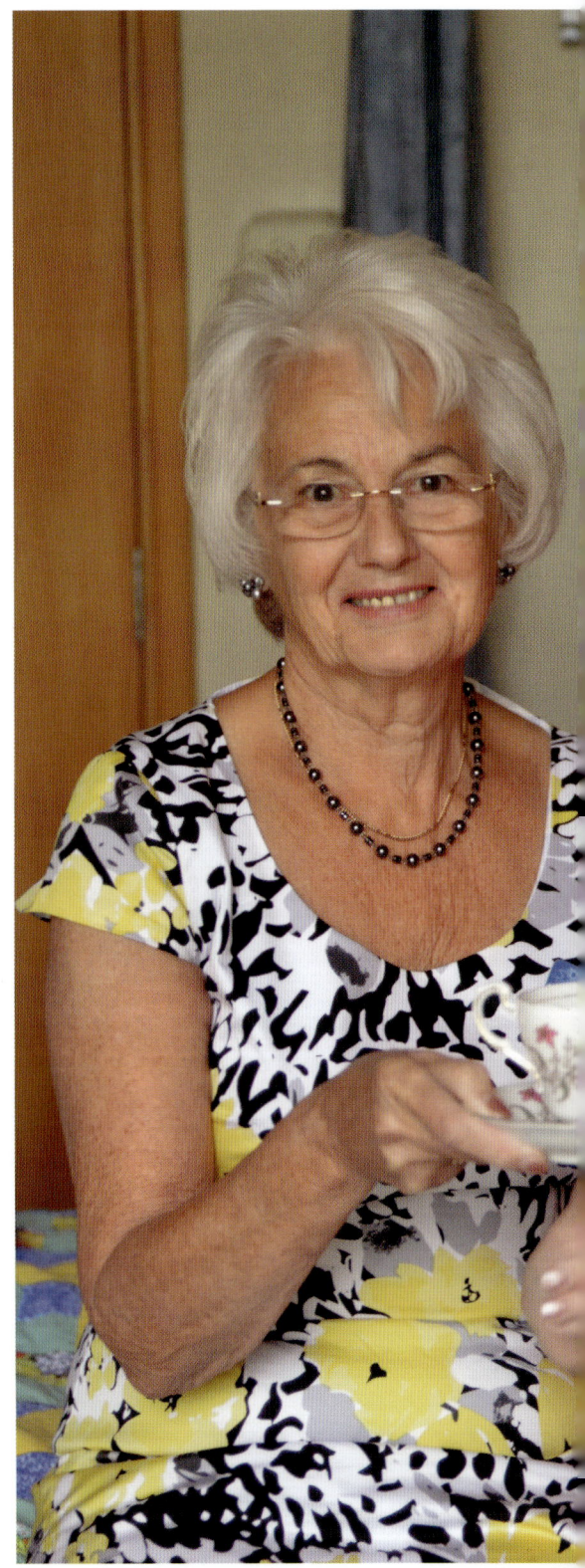

Mum was a founder member of St Michael's Hospice. She worked with the original team at the inception of the hospice; with Freda Pearce, Jeff Kramer and Richard Miller. So St Michael's has always been a part of our lives.

Mum was on Hereford Council and Freda approached her with Jeff and Richard. They had a meeting and it sparked into life. That was at the very, very start. It was close to her heart because she had nursed her own mother during the mid-to-late 1950s, when she was dying of cancer. Mum had to give up her nursing career to look after her own mother, Iris Layton. Her brother also passed away, so she wanted to do something to help people who were in a similar situation to her. Because of those experiences, she realised that more could be done. She was a caring sort. She did a lot for families.

Two of the things that she cared about most were education and social welfare. During her many years on Hereford Council, those were the two things she campaigned about most. So when Freda approached mum about creating a hospice, she just went for it. She was very passionate about it. She was driven to help make it happen.

Mum described herself as being an ambitious and motivated person who strove to make her

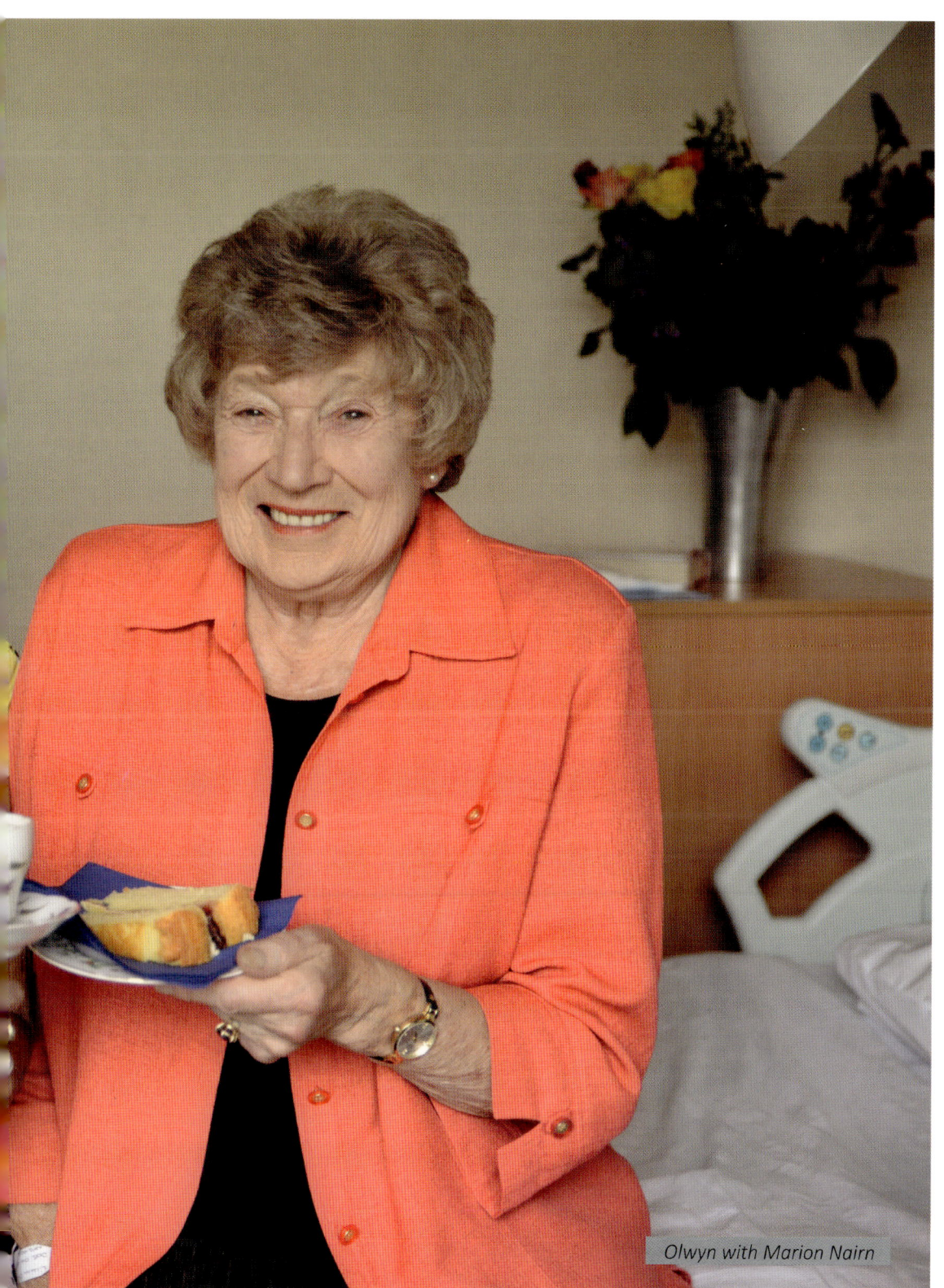

Olwyn with Marion Nairn

own little piece of the world a better place. Those were her words. That's how she described things. I know that she left the initial meeting about the hospice very inspired and St Michael's became a profoundly important part of her life – and ours, too.

When mum had the opportunity, it was a chance for her to embrace things with heart, body and soul. She never doubted for one moment that it wouldn't be achievable. It was just an idea, just a vision when Olwyn got involved.

In the beginning, mum's principle role was to support Freda. Then when St Michael's opened she became vice chairman to Jeff. Then she became chairman. That was right back in the early days, back in the 1980s. She did step back in later life but didn't stop with the fundraising and with her support. She was committed from day one right until the end.

'She put everyone else before her and did a lot for other people.'

When it began, mum was great because she managed to get all of the Hereford people involved. She'd also take Freda out to Powys so that people along the Welsh border became supportive. Mum and Freda were like-minded people, in the sense that if they wanted something done they would get it done. Mum was a strong-minded person. She put everyone else before her and did a lot for other people.

I think I'd have been in my 20s when the hospice all started, I remember it very clearly. The hospice and the council were at the heart of things for mum. But her family was also at the centre of her world. Olwyn was a daughter, wife, mother and grandmother and she made time for everyone.

It might be difficult for some people to understand how determined and devoted mum

was. It sometimes felt as though she'd fit us all in between the letter writing and the phone calls. One thing that was quite funny at the time was this: I used to live not far away and I knew how busy mum was. So on one particular day I rang her up and said: 'I'd like to make an appointment with you'. That became a standing joke. We'd ring her up and ask for an appointment.

And then when we'd get round there, there'd often be a little note on the table from her saying: 'Sorry, had to go out'. But she was just so passionate. With mum, tomorrow was never an option. If it could be done today it would be. That's the sort of person she was. With her passion, motivation and determination, allied to Freda's vision, they made a formidable team. That's how the hospice began. In simple terms, Freda would ask for help with something and it would be up to mum to sort it out. It would be sorting out events and getting people onside, all sorts of things. Between the two of them, with the others, that's what they did.

Before St Michael's, there was no facility in Herefordshire. People would have died in hospital or gone home. They wanted a purpose-built facility where people would be comfortable. Mum believed in equality, respect and commitment. Through the process of fundraising and building the hospice there was never 'I'. It was always 'we', the team. Throughout her life, I watched her win battles. She would fight long and hard when things went wrong. If there were ever problems, she would solve them. If there were challenges, she would embrace them. If there were goals, she would struggle to achieve them. That's my perspective. She would have said things differently; she'd have said she united, discussed,

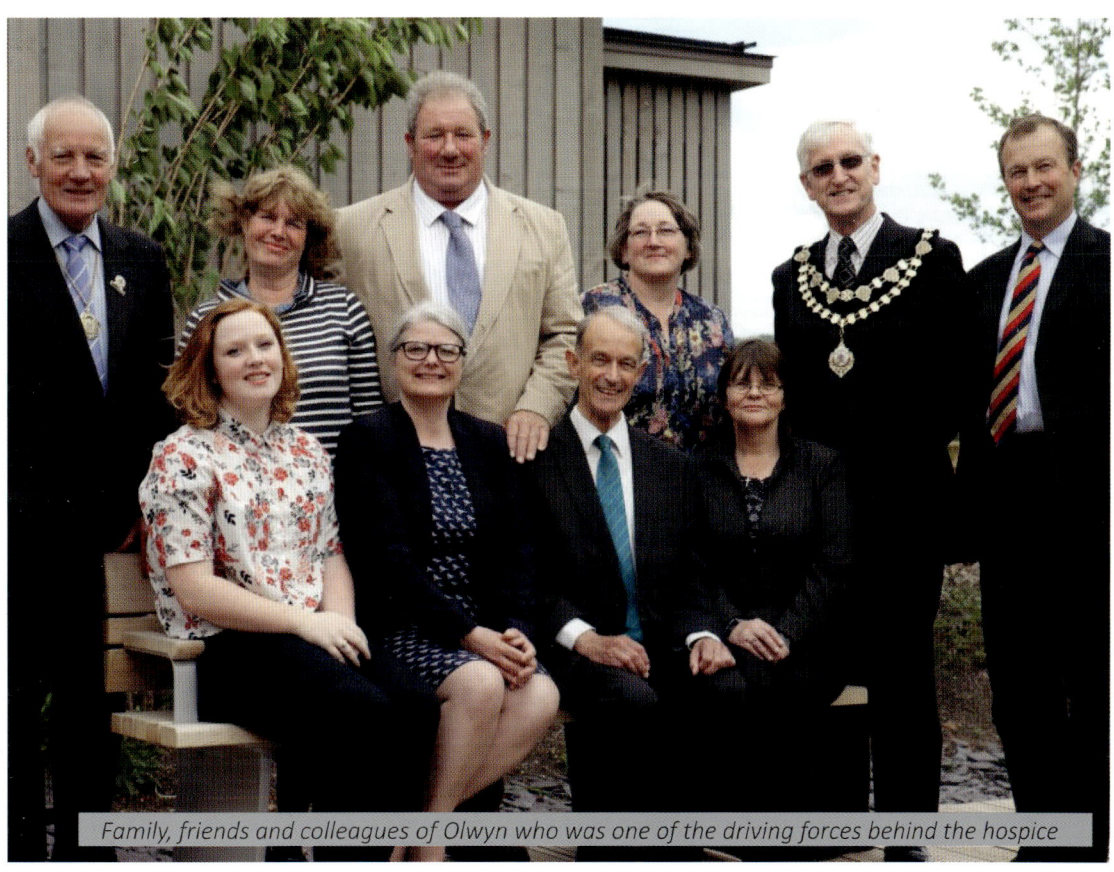

Family, friends and colleagues of Olwyn who was one of the driving forces behind the hospice

delegated and helped. That's how she'd have put it.

Even when she stepped back from the hospice, she didn't step back far. She would always be supporting and fundraising, especially with the new build. Her years as chair were very important to her, I know that. Mum was on so many committees and she achieved near enough every seat there was to hold on Hereford Council. Her commitment to the hospice was unwavering, she stayed the course. She also passed that on to all of us. As a family, all of us take part in events and show our support. Whenever we give to charity, it's always St Michael's. We don't even look at other charities, it's always 100% St Michael's. My niece, for instance, has just done a skydive and raised £700. That went to the hospice. Mum used to have birthday parties; she wouldn't accept any gifts, it was all about donations being made to the hospice.

Mum was the sort of person who once met was never forgotten. She strived. Everything that she approached, she did to the best of her ability and more. And she loved it. I remember asking her once why she was so motivated and happy all the time. She said that every day she would get up in the morning and think of something to smile about before she got out of bed. She said if you wore a smile the world would smile with you. She was a good example to others, simply. I know I'm a little bit biased, but she was a good example of the human race. It didn't matter where you came from or who you were, she'd say that if you respected others they would respect you.

Even opposition councillors on Hereford Council, they all thought she was wonderful. She never followed. She was a leader. The only person she ever followed was Freda, when they worked together for the good of St Michael's. If she put her mind to something, she achieved it. She was just remarkable. When Freda passed away, mum became even more motivated. It was as though she picked up the torch and decided to carry it.

There were other interests in her life, too. She loved dancing, for instance, and she also loved gardening. Her house was immaculate. She'd get up at 4am in the morning in the summer to clean the house, much to our disgust. She'd be Hoovering under our beds by 6.30am to make sure the house was shipshape before she went to work. There were four kids: Philip, Graham, myself and Caroline, then dad, Bill.

Dad worked two jobs and mum did too. Dad worked on the water board and drove a lorry. Mum was a matron, then she was on the council and St Michael's. They weren't lazy. We were all brought up in an old school style. The boys were told to stand tall and walk with their back straight. They always had a pair of clean shoes. Same with us girls, we were taught to respect everybody. It was a good childhood. We were told that we would have everything we needed but not necessarily everything we wanted. We were grateful for what we had and we didn't worry about the things we didn't have.

She loved poetry, too. One of the ones she wrote could easily have been about the people she met at St Michael's. It went:

As I journey along life's path,
There are many paths on which to stray.
The one I'm on just twists and bends
But on it I've found you, my friends.
As I stumble along the path,
It's always you that makes me laugh,
The troubles in which I sometimes land
It's always you that lends a hand.
With all the fun and all the strife
And all the things that make up life,
I thank you for the many ways
In which you help me through the days,
For when my road comes to its end,
That's the thing only heaven knows,
I'll have no regrets that the journey ends,
I love my life because of my friends.

She wrote a lot of poetry. She was articulate.

She was from humble beginnings and they had nothing when they started out. I watched my mum spend hours rubbing down tables in the early days, that's what people did. She would make things. She believed that you should never be either a lender or a borrower. She had those old-fashioned values.

She came to the hospice herself, at the end. She had cancer and was nursed herself.

She came into the hospice to see about her medication and while she was here she did a video called The Extra Mile, it's on YouTube. She had the vision to raise some more money, even though she'd got cancer. She got people together and suggested doing a Christmas Fair. For the first time in my life, I realised that mum was predominantly a delegator. She delegated all the roles to other people. I found it quite funny. In the week she spent as a patient here, she expressed how privileged she'd felt to be part of the hospice for

'Mum was a big believer that it was all about the team'

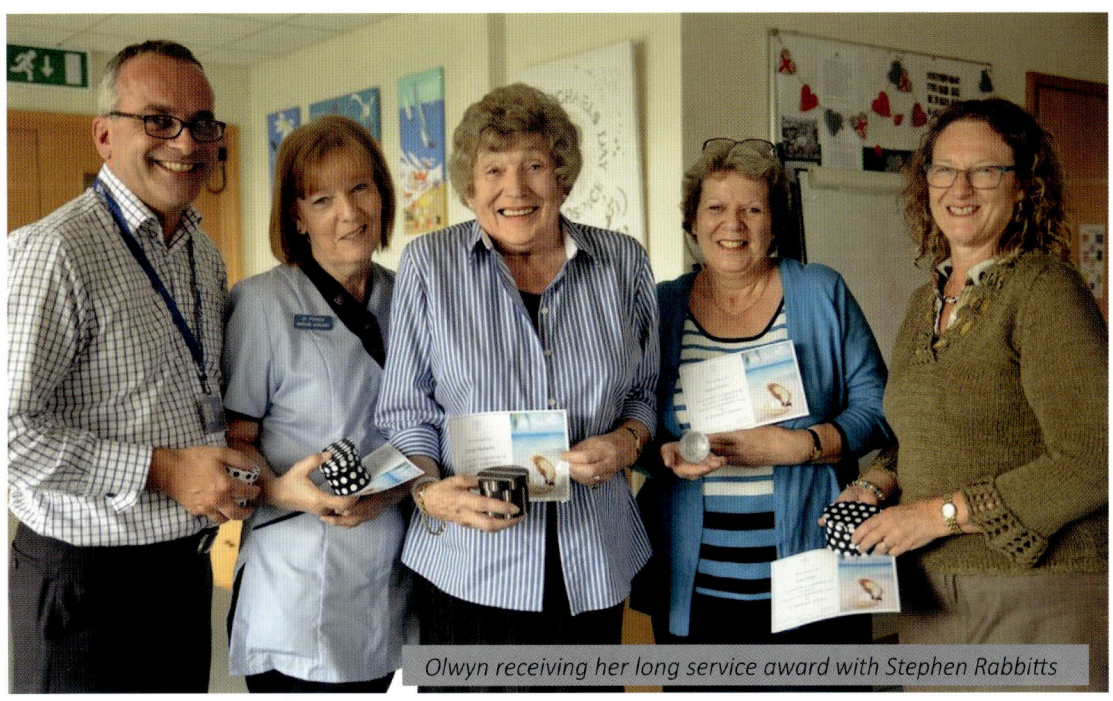

Olwyn receiving her long service award with Stephen Rabbitts

all these years.

She saw two of her relatives die here, too, and that gave her first-hand experience of the quality of the services. Her grandchild, Clare, had been in St Michael's and died, followed very closely by her youngest son, Graham, who had cancer. That happened within 12 months. Mum herself had been battling for a while with cancer, before succumbing. She read the eulogy at her son's funeral and was undaunted. There were two sides to her: there was a public mum and then there was a private mum. It was almost like they were two separate people. She had high expectations of us. She expected us to conduct ourselves properly. She had high standards and expected us to have them too. We found ourselves not doing anything wrong because it would have been disrespectful to our parents if we had.

When mum was ill, it didn't interfere with her schedule at all. She would go to radiotherapy and book the sessions in for 8am so that she could attend meetings in the afternoon. The day before she passed away, she was on the phone still making sure things were in place. She was still organising the Christmas Fair, she was emailing councillors. Her work didn't ever end. She was committed and that's one of the reasons why St Michael's has been so successful. It's been driven by people like Freda and mum. But she was the least boastful person you might meet. She would never take credit for anything. Mum was a big believer that it was all about the team: the volunteer making the tea and the doctor, you need them both. Without them, there would be no hospice.

Barbara Lydia Olive Gwinnell, 64 Ross on Wye

By Rachel Haworth, daughter

I'm sitting at a gorgeous old kitchen table looking across to the Welsh mountains. My journey in reliving this will be tough, but my reasons for wanting to tell my story are greater than any distressing emotions I might feel.

I was born in 1967. My mum was 19. As I grew older, I revelled in the fact that I'd have many years to share my life with her. With only 20 years between us, we were best friends and sisters. There was nothing I couldn't share with her. She and my late dad had a difficult relationship and separated when I was seven. She met my stepfather and stayed with him until the end.

My mum was first diagnosed with ovarian cancer 20 years ago. She was younger than I am now, just 44. Treatments then were not as advanced as they are now; though I hold no resentment about that, just sheer joy that conditions for patients have improved.

At the time, I was living in The Middle East where I was teaching people to wreck-dive and photograph their experience within the power of the seas. I was oblivious that my 'Mur', as I called her, was having the first of many chemotherapy treatments. She had decided to not worry me and would maybe tell me about her fight at a later date. Her tigress-like motherly instincts had kicked in and she wanted to protect me. I began

to understand those instincts later in life, when I became a mother in 2006.

Mur suffered horrendous side effects; severe mouth ulcers, constant sickness, bed sores, hair loss, weakness and more, though she protected me from that.

Some years later, her statutory medical appointments became less frequent and at that point she casually told me that she had had cancer but was now in recovery. She was the mother big cat telling her cub that 'everything was alright'. Her reassurance worked and I didn't worry, after all, she was well again.

Looking back, I now realise she wasn't. My relationship with my stepfather had been tempestuous for many years, though we tolerated each other for Mur's sake. It was not easy; I am told I am a fiery and passionate person, so a benign disposition was difficult to administer.

My Mur was forever by my side. While in labour for 72 hours with my beautiful daughter Poppi, Mur's support was endless. The number of calls to the delivery suite was huge. Eventually, I shouted: 'Please tell my mum to go to bed'. When Poppi eventually put in her appearance, Mur and my stepfather came to visit. Poor Poppi's father was exhausted, but remained a tower of support. Mur came in on her own while I was feeding Poppi. She said: 'Oh dear, I think I may cry'. It was a rare moment of emotion. Mur did not cry very often in front of me, she was always incredibly thoughtful and brave, but that moment touched her more deeply than I could have imagined.

Mur was delighted for me. She only wished for my happiness and peace. When she held Poppi for the first time, I photographed it.

It was near to Christmas and soon we took Poppi home for the first time. Mur fell deeper and deeper with a Grandparent's precious love and she and Poppi became the very best of friends. As Poppi grew towards three years old, we spoke of plans for her to attend a nursery school near to

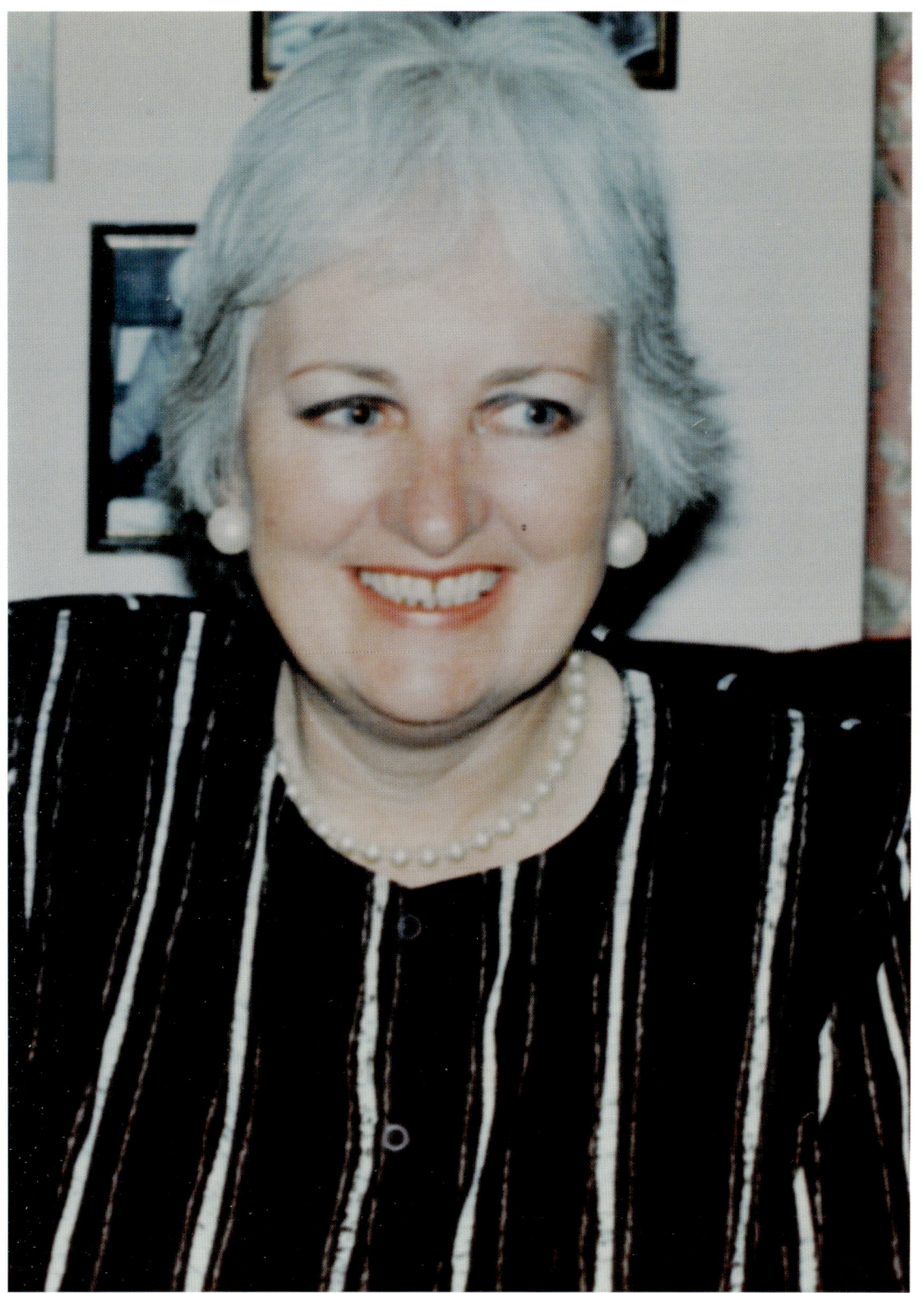

where Mur lived, just so that she could see more of her. Mur's bungalow was filled with Poppi's toys and photographs. Her handbag was also swimming with treats and a Proud Grandma Book. Life was good, very good.

A knock on the door some three years later changed my life more dramatically than anything I have ever experienced. Life rocked me to my feet in an instance.

Mur and my stepfather stood at the doorstep, serious expressions crowding their faces. They never turned up without calling ahead.

Immediately, I sensed something grave. Mur held Poppi and very calmly explained to me that the cancer had returned but that she was going to have treatment.

I worried deeply about Mur. I made a conscious decision not to Google cancer and I avoided reading about it. It was a very confusing time. How could the cancer return when she'd had her ovaries removed? Naively, or more likely, taking an ostrich-like, head-in-the-sand stance, I refused to accept that everything would not be alright. Mur was unconquerable and invincible; she would have to be alright.

Mur decided to have a very special hair appointment. She knew she would lose her hair again so she treated herself to a pampering. Her treatment began and on her first session at The Charles Renton unit, in Hereford, I appeared with Poppi in my arms to wish her well. I didn't go in with her, I didn't want to nor did she want me to.

Many treatments followed over the next two years; Mur relishing the energy-giving effects of the steroids immediately afterwards. They enabled her to get lots of things done before the next lull in her immune system took its toll.

My love for her seemed to grow stronger and each year I arranged major birthday presents.

On one occasion, I arranged to have her collected by helicopter to fly over the Black Mountains and The Sugar Loaf in Wales, where her mother had lived. I wanted to spoil her, it was the least she deserved.

But Mur's decline was inexorable. Her health became progressively worse and she gradually became unable to walk far without becoming breathless.

Not that her spirit was defeated. The reverse was true. She never once complained. She kept being the perfect mother that she had always been. To Mur, cancer was almost an inconvenience, it was secondary to her life and she refused to let it beat her. The word 'secondary', however, came to haunt me because secondary cancers were the reason for her decline.

During the 11th of 12 chemotherapy sessions, Mur began to discuss the happiness of her blood counts improving.

'She never once complained. She kept being the perfect mother that she had always been.'

Our wonderful friend, Poppi's godmother, Sue, would collect Mur. She would be armed with a hot water bottle to keep Mur's veins fat as they became increasingly un-co-operative with hospital needles. Mur's journey to hospital was made more comfortable by a soft blanket, a flapjack and her favourite music. Mur would actively look forward to Sue's company and those comfortable journeys. The two of them formed an incredible bond and Sue remains a rock to us still.

My own life became increasingly busy and around that time I was due to conduct my first

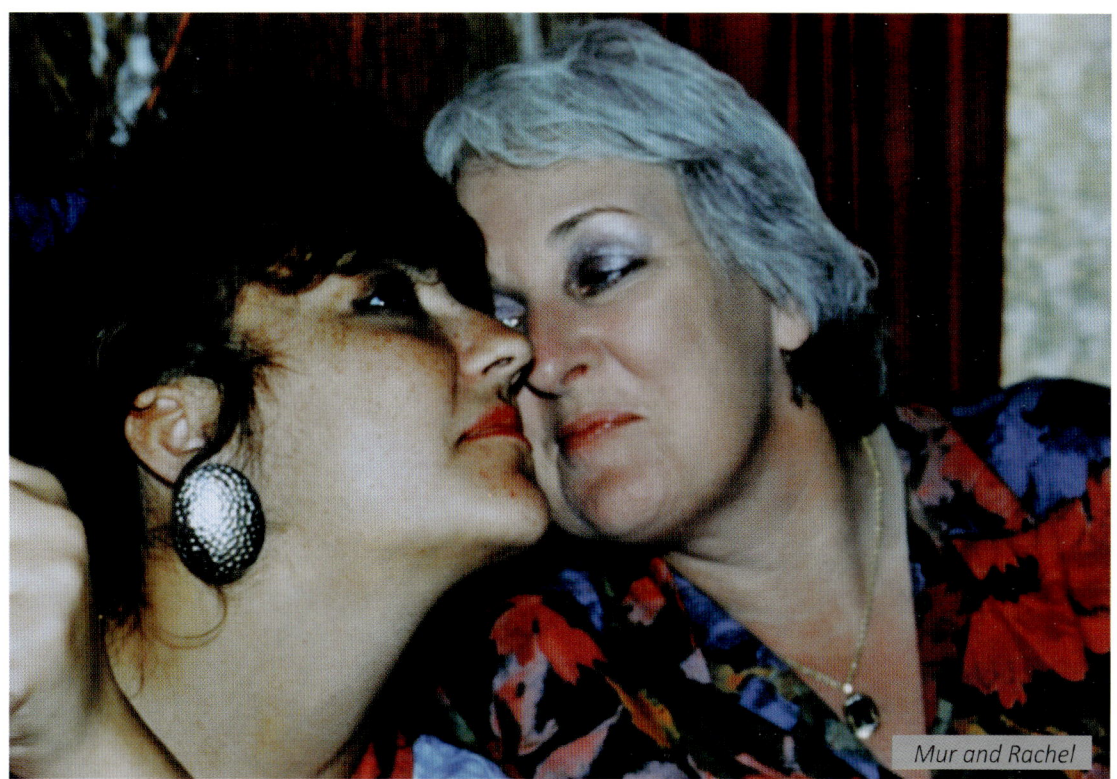

Mur and Rachel

cookery demonstration. Mur was deeply thrilled and told me that she thought I would develop more in that area. I was nervous about what lay in store but Mur calmed my nerves. As I drove towards The Sugar Loaf she softly assured me that everything would be okay. 'But Mur, what if I run out of things to say?' She laughed, knowing that I had never run out of things to say.

My demonstration came and was a hit. People loved it and I felt on top of the world. But little did I know that an ambulance had been called for Mur. She had been taken to hospital. I received a text from her afterwards: 'Well, how did it go?' I called her home number, to talk, but there was no answer. It was December and Mur had been taken to hospital.

Mur was admitted to an oncology unit in Cheltenham. She had developed pneumonia. I went to see her but she was in a poor condition, hooked up to many tubes and machines and heavily sedated. There were too few staff and Mur had been hallucinating. She was uncomfortable and it was distressing to see her being inexpertly cared for. Mur had earlier made a decision that if her 12 treatments were unsuccessful, she would discontinue. She had no appetite for further treatment. The programme had become futile.

Mur's regime was to change. Palliative care nurses were called and they calmly sat with us around Mur's bed and told he that her life was close to an end. The news left me shocked, though Mur remained calm. Typically, her thoughts were for the nurses, rather than herself. 'What a difficult job they have,' she said. Her spirit, however, had not been defeated. 'But I will decide when I go, not the medical profession'.

The palliative care team was unsure whether Mur would have days or a week. They did, however, know that her time was short and that it would not extend to months.

I had heard about St Michael's Hospice and I fought to get a transfer there. The oncology unit at Cheltenham was ill-equipped to cope and I needed her to be in more comfort and enjoy a better quality of life. My campaigning yielded poor results; St Michael's Hospice was full and another hospice in Wales was also full.

I refused to give in and soon the palliative care team informed me that a room was available in Bartestree. St Michael's Hospice had made it happen.

I was filled with dread by Mur's admission to St Michael's. Like many people, my preconceived idea of a hospice was completely wrong. I had imagined Mur would be entering a cabbage-smelling death house. I could not have been more wrong.

When I arrived at St Michael's I was greeted by the kindest gentleman on the reception, who immediately put me at ease. I was in an obvious state of agitation and each member of staff spoke to me, helping to bring calm. I was grateful beyond words that Mur wasn't in a hell hole.

Mur's improvement was immediately apparent. For the first time in days, she was brighter. She was still unable to walk but she was chatty and even a little hungry. The nurses asked what Mur would like, which I found incredible after our earlier experience elsewhere. She ordered porridge made with cream and brown sugar. 'It's beautiful,' she told me. There was a visitor's room where drinks could be made and a peaceful refuge in which I could reflect and take time to adjust.

I visited as often as I could and my heart never once stopped pounding as I drove along the hospice road. My only focus was on spending as much quality time with Mur as I could.

The relationship between my stepfather and I was difficult, but the hospice staff realised things were amiss and helped to enable meaningful visits. Their only objective was that Mur should have the best care.

Grief affects people differently but I refused to let the difficulties undermine my time with Mur. She was moved to a bed beside glass doors, which overlooked apple orchards. And she found happiness there. The doctors took a number of decisions to improve Mur's care and I was allowed precious uninterrupted time with her. I will never be able to thank the hospice enough for being so sensitive towards my family. Their actions completely changed my perceptions and I will forever be grateful.

Mur was able to spend time with my daughter, Poppi, too. They lifted one another's spirits immeasurably. Poppi would walk the short distance with Mur to the bathroom. My daughter would walk slowly and methodically with Mur, who was supported by a frame. They would hold hands, best friends forever, and I observed several staff stopping in their tracks to smile. The moment was dear and remains so.

In February 2012, Mur was allowed to leave the hospice. She had surpassed the 'few days or weeks' that had been given to her. She was thrilled about going home and, stupidly, I imagined she might get better. As she walked with her frame, she hugged staff. They gave her a round of applause for resisting a wheelchair as she made her way to the exit. The relationship with St Michael's continued and staff offered support in all areas, with additional help at home and care.

Though the following month was fraught, we made the best of the time we had. When Mother's Day arrived in March, I arranged lunch. Mur and I were in the brightest pink outfits and she discussed Easter bunnies with Poppi. We even had a few photographs together, the last that were taken.

Just 10 days later, I was called to Hereford County Hospital at 6am. I was told to come quickly because Mur had fallen from her bed. I

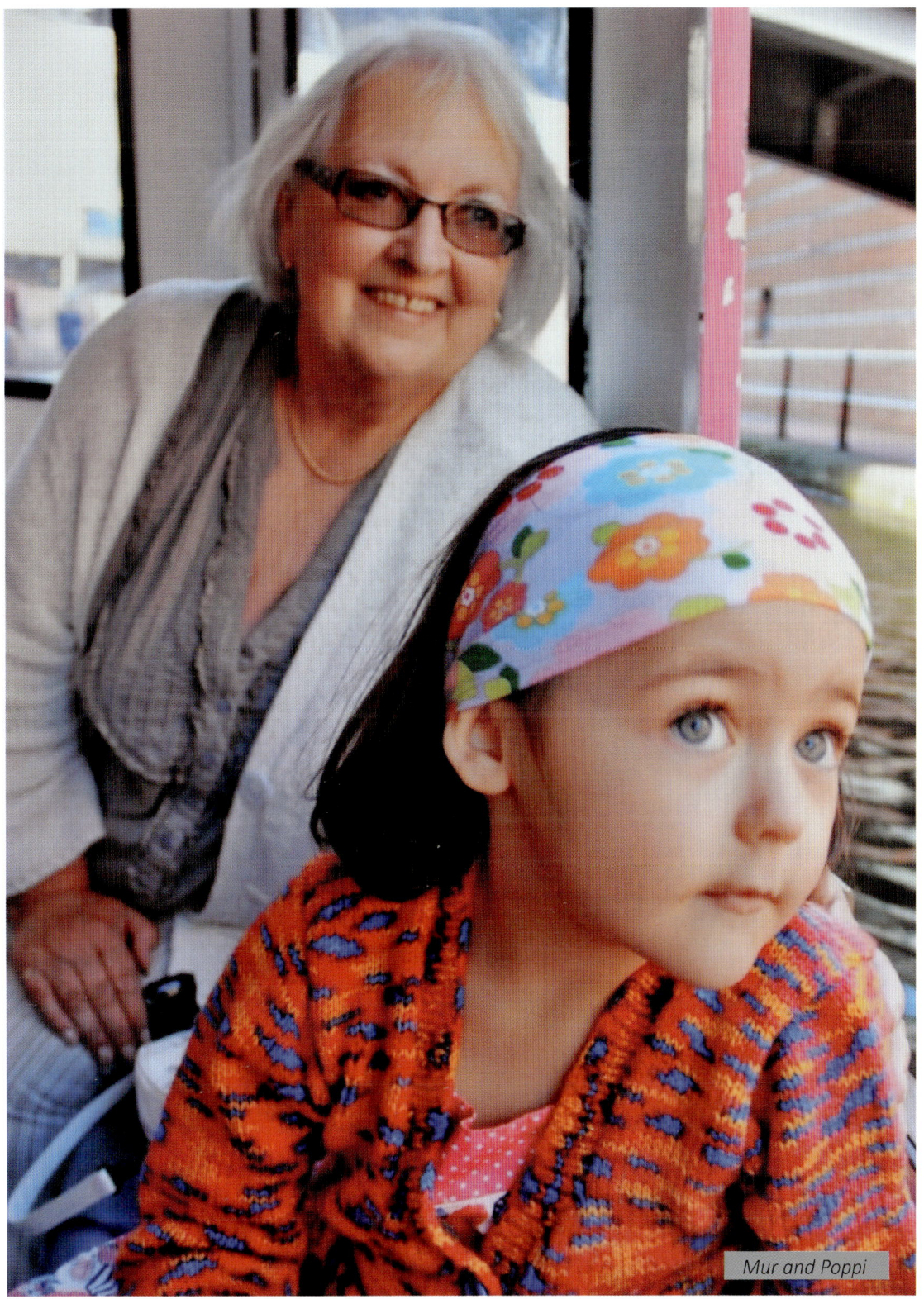

Mur and Poppi

was greeted by a hard, tiny Scottish nurse, who explained that my mother looked very poorly and had been taken for a scan. I, meanwhile, went to see two doctors who told me that Mur was nearing the end of her life. I knew that they were right this time; my Mur had decided, as she'd told us all, that very soon we must let her go.

I held her hand and her eyes stayed open. I was told that she still might be able to hear me, although she was gravely ill.

In those final days, I enjoyed special moments with Mur. On occasions, she felt a little better. I remember walking towards her bed and observing that she was alone, eating a yoghurt, sitting in a bedside chair. She was so pleased to see me and gave me a gardening magazine, knowing how poor my gardening skills were. At night, I would sent her a text, as I always did: 'Night Night Mur xx'. I avoided using the word 'goodnight' because it felt so final. I would end by telling her about something that Poppi had done and I would wish her wonderful dreams.

The Gods have a peculiar way of moving through our lives and when the end neared, I instinctively knew. A white feather landed on my foot and with it came an overwhelming urge to be with Mur.

I took the bull by the horns and armed with a few wonderful close friends of mum, I went to her.

She had changed dramatically, I had never seen anyone dying before and was quite shocked at how the colour of life seems to disappear before the heartbeat stops. I was in a terribly emotional state, I held her hand and said 'It'll be alright Mur'.

How the tables had turned, there was I telling my mum the very words she had used to me.

Within seconds she took her last breath. She had waited for me. I kept the feather.

During the next few months and after the funeral the disbelief of it all was great. My stepfather passed away three days after mum's funeral. His health was not good and had not been for many years.

I attended a bereavement support group at the hospice. It was an emotional but therapeutic time. The staff were absolutely professional and incredibly understanding. The support continued and I met one of their highly trained volunteers every few months over a two-year period. My wonderful support volunteer was a retired doctor and during that period he helped me to face the demons and devils of grief. He could see how difficult things had been and helped me to see things more clearly.

I remember the first time he came to the house, I had never experienced counselling of any kind before and was very uncomfortable. Within seconds I was in floods of tears, a common factor during those two years with that saint of a man.

On the last occasion, we sort of realised that it was time to go it alone. We shook hands and he told me that I could contact him at any time, the help and support would never leave me.

And that is one of my abiding thoughts about St Michael's: It never abandons people. It reminds me of a quote from the movie Nanny Mcphee. 'If you need me, but do not want me, I will stay. If you want me, but no longer need me then I have to go'. Those words summed up how I felt.

The hospice helped me reach the path of acceptance. When the doctor and I shook hands on that day, my heart was filled with fear at the thought that there would be no more meetings, though the option for them still remains open.

The idea for 20 Beds was born at the same Welsh table that I'm sitting at now, writing about Mur. I know that I would never have come this far without the help I received from that incredible and unbelievable establishment. It provided a quality of life for my Mur that I had thought inconceivable. And it supported me, as an individual, more than I could have imagined.

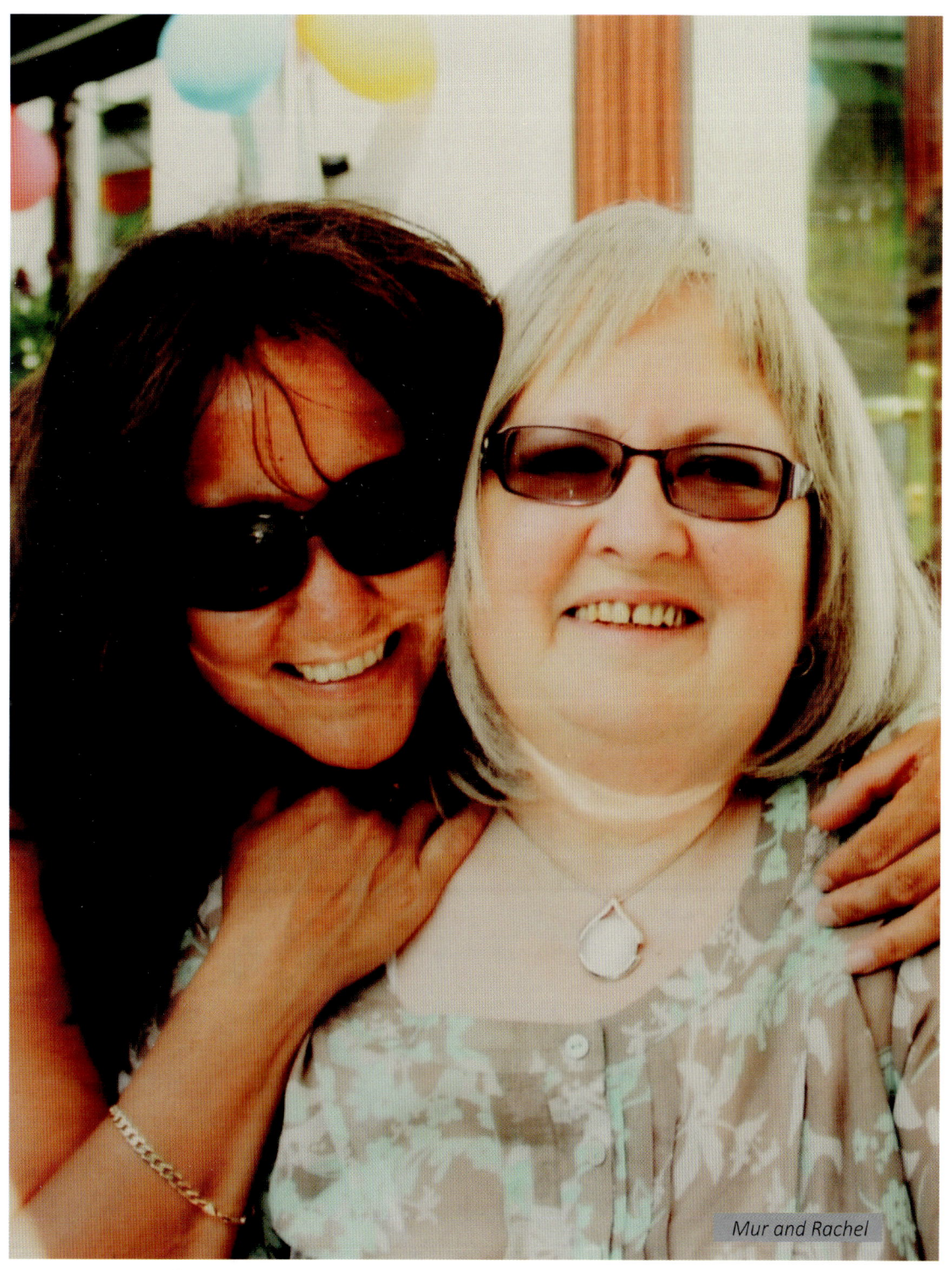

Mur and Rachel

Russell Sharp, 48 Llandrindod Wells

I've always been a happy-go-lucky guy. I've led a colourful life. There have been ups and downs – and in my case I've probably had more than most. But that's part of life's rich tapestry, isn't it. Our experiences are what make us who we are.

I've had time to reflect on my life during the past four months; that's how long I've been here, at St Michael's Hospice. It's the middle of summer now – July 31st, since you ask – and I was admitted at the start of April.

I'm 48, that's all, 48. I should be in the prime of my life. But I'm bed-bound, unable even to walk. I've got two months to live, or so the doctors tell me.

Things started to go wrong just before Christmas. I went to the toilet on a Friday morning and stayed there for four hours. I was in agony. I know it sounds disgusting, and I'm sorry if it does, but that's when things started to unravel. I had to call an ambulance and they rushed me into Hereford Hospital. They told me almost straight away: 'I'm sorry, Mr Sharp, we think you may have cancer. We're going to send you for more tests'.

They found it when they were cleaning me up. It was a bolt from the blue. I didn't realise anything was wrong. I was diagnosed soon after.

The biopsies confirmed that I'd got anal cancer. It was pretty severe, the doctor told me it was the worst case in the country. I struggled on at home for a while, I'll tell you about that in a minute, as well as some of the stories from my life.

In spring, I couldn't go on any more; the pain was too intense. So I came to St Michael's. I was told I'd got six months to live and so far I've had four. I just get on with it, what else can you do?

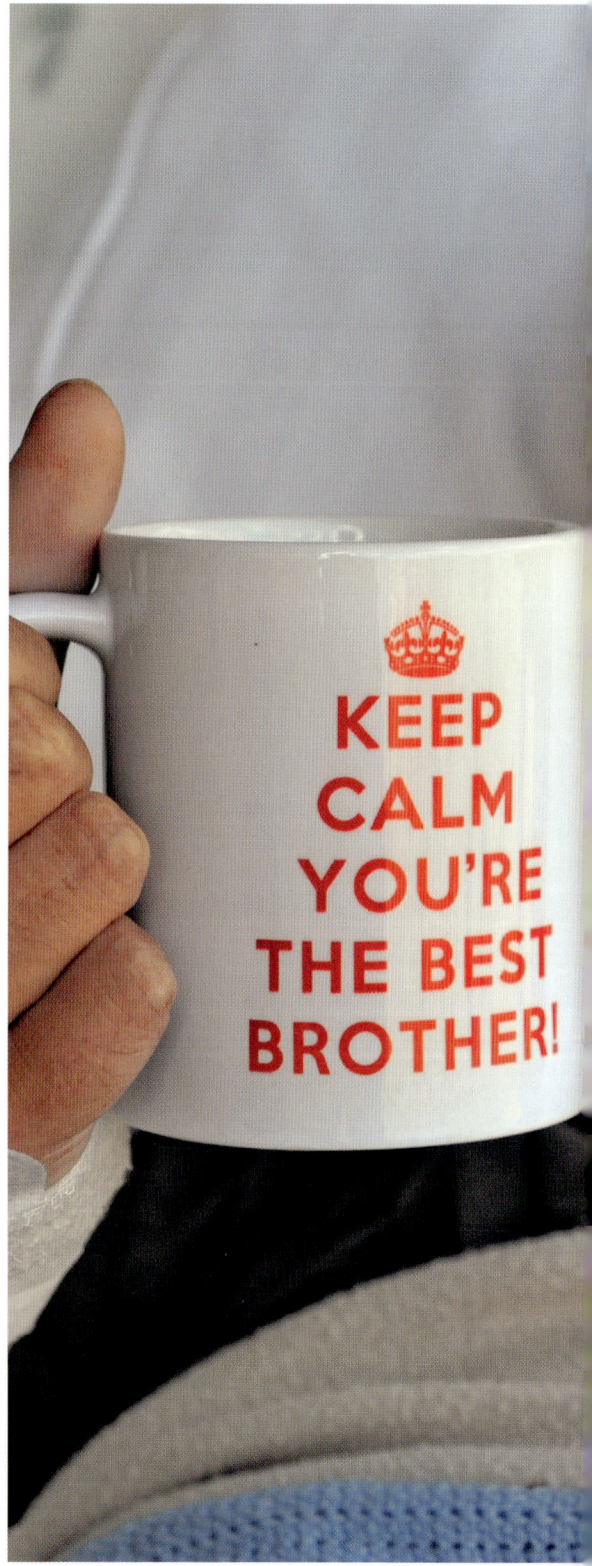

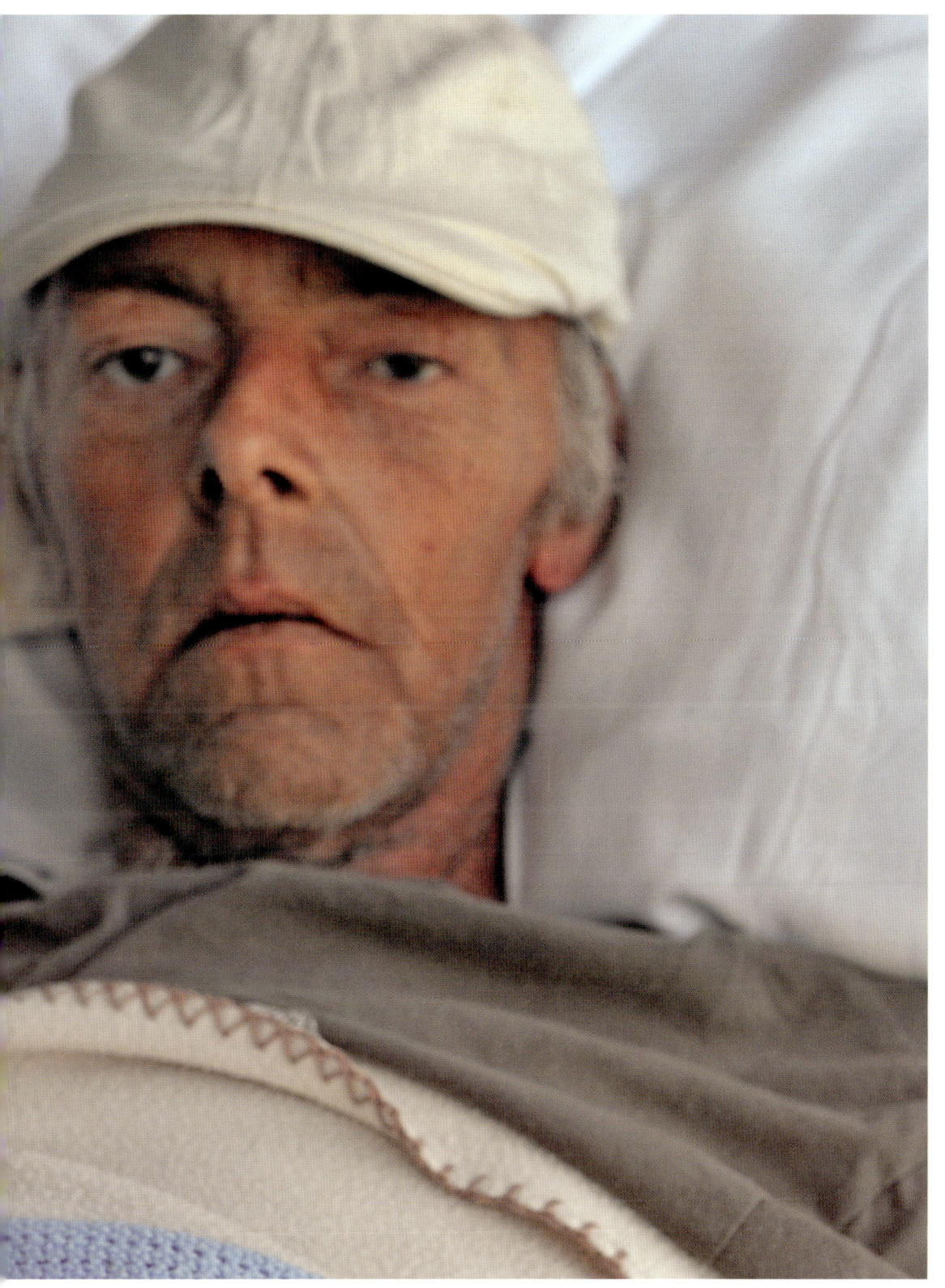

I'd have liked to have stayed at home, in Llandrindod Wells, for longer. But the pain was too much and I couldn't even sit down. Now I can't do anything, I can't walk because I've lost the use of my legs. Half of that's my own fault because I refused to get out of bed. I had a nerve block on my right side, about a month ago. Some of the nerves have been killed in my right leg. We were supposed to be working on that to get the feeling back, so that I could walk again. But one day I just told them I'd had enough, I couldn't do it. And that's where I am now.

At one point, I thought I might be shipped out to the hospital at Llandrindod Wells. But they let me stay here at the hospice, which is much better.

I'm supposed to only have two months left, but I can see myself going on for longer than that. I should be ill now. I mean I'm ill, yes. You can see that. You can tell by looking at my photo, too. But I'm fine, you know. I'm okay. I'm nowhere near as ill as I should be. I'm nowhere near as ill as they expected. I feel alright. I'll keep going for a while yet; it will be for longer than they said. I could go downhill like a rocket between now and September but I can't see it, myself. I'm going to stick around for a while yet.

I was at home when I got ill. I'd started up a hobby, making doll's houses. I was making them with pieces of timber. Wooden houses, they were. But in the end I had to stop doing that because I couldn't stand long enough to do it. I was making them and selling them. I'd only just started up. I'd bought £1,000 worth of furniture for them, I was buying off ebay every day and I was the best one on the site. But that went out the window as soon as I got ill.

Nothing can prepare you for suddenly falling ill.

The day that I fell ill was just like any other. It was a humdrum Friday, nothing unusual. And then all hell broke loose.

Within 48 hours I was being examined; they put a camera up, which was really horrible. By the Tuesday, I was having biopsies and on the Thursday they gave me my formal diagnosis; although they knew from day one.

Imagine that happening, all in the space of a week.

One minute you are fine and by the evening you've been rushed into hospital and you're being told you've probably got cancer.

Within two days, they're carrying out tests and then another two days later, you're being told it may be over. It's frightening.

I'm just a normal guy. I'll do anything for anybody, to a certain point, y'know. I didn't think anything was wrong with me on the Friday, well, nothing serious. I was even ordering new furniture off ebay on the Friday, when I first went in. I assumed everything would be alright. I didn't think there'd be any reason to stop. I just thought it was a bad day, y'know. I just thought: 'get on with it'.

I must have spent £500 on parts, furniture and another doll's house while I was in hospital. I didn't think I had anything to worry about.

I've been married before, but I was living alone when I got ill. I had a flat in Llandrindod Wells. I

'I'm supposed to only have two months left . . . but I can't see it myself. I'm going to stick around for a while yet.'

was by myself. I don't have any kids, which I'm grateful for, because that would have been too painful for everyone now.

At first, I thought it was just something that happens. I was going to just get on with it. I kept asking how long I'd got left. They wouldn't answer me because they didn't know. It upset me a bit, y'know.

Every day was getting worse and worse. It was more and more painful to sit down.

So I ended up lying down all the time. I would just be on my side. Then the pain just got that much I couldn't stand it anymore so I ended up coming in here. I had my last Christmas at home but things went downhill after that and by April I was in the hospice.

I was called in by the consultant and he had a look, examined me, and I asked him how long I'd got.

He said: "Six months, at the most." That really hit me between the eyes.

It got to my brother, Carl, too. He took off like a scalded rat. He just ran out the room, which was quite funny. He was in the room with me and so were all my friends, as well as my sister-in-law. They came with me when I got my diagnosis. Then he came back in the room. It had frightened him. I had a talk to him to calm him down. I got him by himself and explained to him that there was nothing I could do about it. I asked his wife to look after him because he is stressed and I worry that he'll explode. He's stressed all the time. He's a good man.

My best friend was there with me too. She started bawling, so did I. We had a heart-to-heart in the car park then I went to find my brother.

He seemed to have calmed down by then. I just hugged him and told him I was alright. He's younger than me.

Nobody prepares you for the news that you're going to die. You don't know how you're going to react until it happens.

I'm 48 now, so it's a shock to me that I've got cancer. I'm still young. You don't normally hear about these things until people are 50 or 60 but I've got it now. What I don't understand is how I've got it. But they say it lies dormant in everybody. It lies dormant until it's upset.

So the day I went to the toilet is the day the cancer got annoyed and woke up, that's what I think. That was back in October or November, it was certainly well before Christmas.

I try to count my blessings. I'm grateful for being at the hospice, for instance. It's an absolutely fantastic place. They can't do enough for you. I've got my own room, with a telly. They wheel my bed out of the room each day, so that I'm in the sunshine on a patio. It's amazing.

'I try to count my blessings. I'm grateful for being at the hospice, for instance. It's a fantastic place.'

It's peaceful and quiet. I can be outside and still watch my telly.

The nurses call me now and again but they know I'm alright. I love being outside.

I used to be a forklift driver, then we all got laid off from that. That was out in Wales. The place where I worked closed down. Then I was in-between jobs and making the doll's houses to keep busy. And then I got ill.

I'm going to be honest with you. There's no reason not to be. It's important to tell you these things because one day they might help somebody else. They might reassure somebody else that they're not alone, that other people get ill too.

At first, the worst thing was the pain. I coped between October until December. But at Christmas, it all got too much.

The pain, wow, I've never had pain like it, never. It was all day and all night. The pain was out of the ballpark. I put up with it for a while but then I came here, to the hospice. I had a breakdown not long after coming here because the pain was too much. They were giving me painkillers, but I was fighting those as well as the pain.

One day, I collapsed when I was in my room. I went out like a light. I was doing something and the nurses were with me. I said to one of the nurses: 'I'm going down'. And she knew what I meant, somehow. She moved round and stood behind me. Then I went down. It took four of them to get me up.

They haven't told me a lot and I can't remember anything else about it.

Apparently my brother was here. And he reckons I was fighting the nurses like a cat. I was really fighting them, but I can't remember. I was shouting and swearing at them, apparently. But I can't remember any of it. I haven't a clue, not a bloody clue.

So I ended up having to apologise to them all. It was a bad day, a really bad day and night. The next thing I knew it was the early hours of Tuesday morning. I don't know what I did. I didn't know anything about it, nothing at all. That all happened on the Sunday night. I was supposed to go to Cheltenham Hospital on the Monday, but that was cancelled. I can't remember anything

until the Tuesday.

Before I came to the hospice, I'd had radiotherapy and chemotherapy to try and fight the tumour.

I had radiotherapy for a week, then chemotherapy on top of that in the second week. Then I had chemo for five or six weeks. I had the maximum dose of radiotherapy. I had the top dose. When I had my consultation, they told me that was it. They couldn't do any more for me. Then I had another consultation and they told me that the radiotherapy had stopped working after the first week. But they didn't know that at first. They couldn't work out why it had been unsuccessful, they only knew that it was.

To be honest with you, after the radiotherapy I was bouncing off the walls. I was supposed to be flat on my back in bed, ill. But I was as high as a kite after I'd had it. I was as happy as Larry; you couldn't keep me down.

Any other person would have been ill. That's one of the reasons why it stopped working. I should have been ill but I wasn't.

I was called in for a consultation and they told me the radiotherapy wasn't working. They didn't know why. They didn't know that it had stopped working. At that point, I thought they'd be able to sort me out and get me well. In the second consultation, I was told I'd got six months to live. That really knocked me about for a bit. I was told there was nothing they could do to help.

I was devastated. I had to sort all my stuff out about my flat.

I've got exactly two months left from today. I

> 'I'm just getting on with it now. There's nothing else I can do really. I'd love to be able to get up and walk around.'

won't say I'm counting the time.

I'm counting it in months, though, not days. I can't walk around now but I feel fine. The medication makes me thirsty all the time and I do get occasional pain, I get a kick now and again. But I'm just getting on with it now. There's nothing else I can do really. I'd love to be able to get up and walk around and go places.

When I knew I'd got six months, I just wanted to get on with life and enjoy it. But I can't. But that's why this place is great. I can just be here, by myself, and there's peace and quiet.

My bed is outside during the day and I can lie there and practically watch the leaves grow. I'm surrounded by foliage. I actually see how much things grow each day. I know it might sound like that's just in my imagination, but I can see them grow. It makes me happy. The staff and the facilities? Well, what can I say, I'd give them A plus plus.

I've had time to remember the key moments of my life. I was born in Shrewsbury. I can't remember where. I was there until I was one, then we moved down to Knighton. We lived there for 20-odd years. Then I met the girl next door, literally.

Her mum moved to Weymouth, so we went there too. Then after 18 months, her mum moved back, so we had to move back to. I think that's what spoiled things for us, we shouldn't have moved back. It caused a bit of friction.

Then I met a girl from the other side of the car park, in Knighton. I know that sounds funny, but that's what happened. We got on well. I divorced my first wife and moved in with the new one.

> 'My bed is outside during the day and I can lie there and practically watch the leaves grow. It makes me happy.'

Then she got fed up, she got bored. She pulled the plug on me and chucked me out, so I had to find my own place, which I did. Then there were problems. The police got involved. The whole thing sent me loopy. I moved to Llanfair Caereinion, near Newtown, just to get some peace.

Then I got in trouble. I set fire to my flat and got arrested. I did it on purpose. I got done for arson with intent to endanger my own life. I was charged and sent down for 18 months, but I only did nine. I did it because I was unhappy. I was on a downer, a serious downer. I'd wanted to kill myself. I'd been on my deathbed more than once. I overdosed. The psychiatrist said if I hadn't had snapped out of what I did when I started the fire, I'd have stayed in there and gone up with it.

I phoned the fire brigade and they came. I got the neighbours out, too, that's why I only got intent to endanger my own life. I got the others out so they weren't hurt.

The flat was gutted, I did a very good job of it. I just threw a fag on the settee and let it go. It didn't take long for it to go up.

You know what these settees are like. It was an old settee anyway, so it was probably not fire-proofed.

I went to Mold Crown Court. Then I was sent to Liverpool for nine months. It was like Butlins; I understood why they called it Butlins. I kept my nose clean and made sure everybody else knew that I wanted to keep my nose clean.

Don't get me wrong, I had my first fight the first day I was there. Somebody wanted to prove a point but he picked on the wrong lad. I only hit him once, he went straight down. There were screws round me and him. All the other lads were in there. He walked up to me and took a swing and missed. I said to him: 'my turn now, is it?' I swung, caught him on the end of his jaw, and he went down like a sack of potatoes. I had some power behind me, well, I did.

Everybody laughed at him. He was supposed to be halfway up the scale but he went to the bottom; he was a wimp then.

I weighed 20 stone at the time. I was huge. I had to turn sideways to go through the door.

That's another way that I realised I was ill. The weight just dropped off me. After being consulted, I started losing weight like mad. I was still eating the same things as normal, if not even more, because I knew I had to keep my strength up. And then the weight fell off me. I was on extra supplements to keep my weight up but it just started to drop off me. I went from 20 stone to 12 stone in a month or so. I was down to 10 stone, my weight halved. I like big t-shirts anyway, so I don't mind.

When I was in jail, during the day I just did work in the gym. I built myself up. I was really big. There was a lad in there, Peter Poole, and he was muscle bound. He couldn't put his hands down his sides. And I was as big as him. Peter never told me why he was in. Some of the lads in nick kept their mouths shut on what they've done, which was only fair. But I told them why I was in and then they seemed to keep away a bit more.

They wouldn't let me go back to my old place so I went to Llandrindod Wells, in a hostel. I would have been about 40 or 41. The women were out of my life and I was quite happy.

I found a flat, but it was too cold in the winter so I moved to another place. That's where I was when I got diagnosed.

They look after me fantastically well here. I stay in my room in the hospice. I could go out if I wanted to but I'm quite happy just being in my room and going out into the garden, in my bed.

I'm glad I'm in here and not a hospital, a hospital would be totally different.

Here, I've got my own room. I draw a bit, too, I do a bit of doodling. A place like this makes a big difference to my life, what's left of it. I'm lucky to be here. I still smoke, they let me roll my own when my bed's outside.

I'm a fighter. I battle on. I don't just give up. The nurses come and make sure I'm alright, but once they know I'm fine they'll leave me until something needs doing.

It's nice to have my own space. This place is good. If I want anything, all I have to do is shout.

I sleep every night, more than I used to at home. At home I had pain, I couldn't get comfortable and I couldn't sleep. Here, I'm alright.

I miss driving, that's the worst thing. I miss my car. I can't walk so I can't drive either. I used to just get my car and go for a drive. There were a lot of places around Llandrindod Wells. I'd go up to Rhayader dams, that was one place. Then I'd go up the back road to Aberystwyth and then come back a different route. I'd just enjoy the drive.

I used to love being mobile, I'd enjoy the scenery and stop to take photos. I'd hit the road.

If I wanted a coffee, I'd stop at a roadside café. Sometimes I'd eat there too. I'd stop off, light up and chill out. That was the good thing about it.

Before this happened, I was as free as a bird. And sometimes, when I'm lying outside and the sun is shining, I think I still am.

———————————

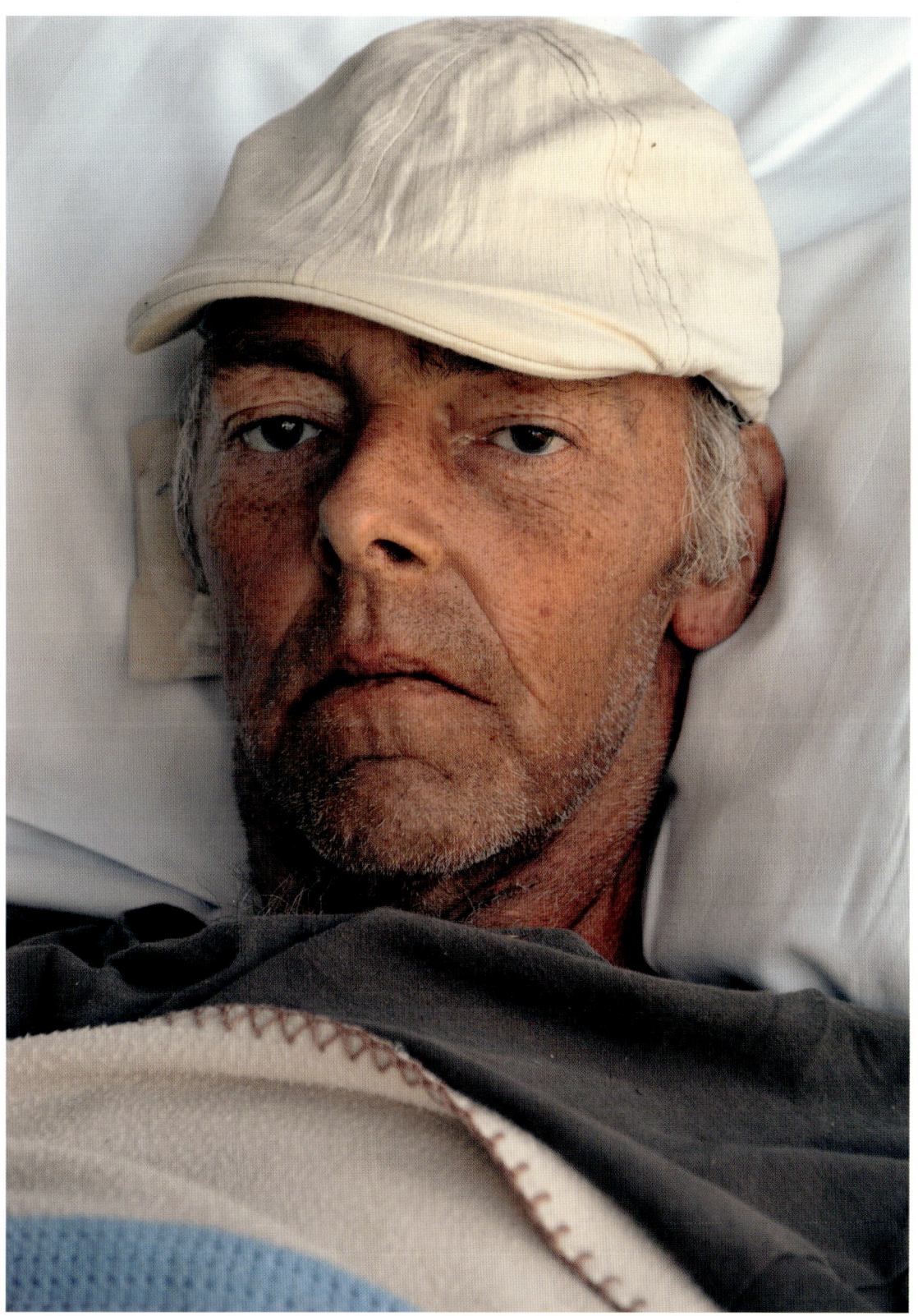

Dotty Cheetham, 95 Holme Lacy

I come to the hospice every Friday. I've been coming for about two months. It's good to come here, it helps me get around. If I'm at home, I don't get to see that much. So being here gives me something different to do, it gives me something interesting during the day and makes me feel happy.

I've been on my own for 30 years now, since my husband died. I live with my son and his family, but I still think about my husband every day. It's a long time ago but I miss him still, definitely.

Robert was his first name. He was wounded very badly in the War. He had shrapnel in his spine and suffered an awful lot. I looked after him as well as I could. I had him in a wheelchair for seven months before he died.

We were both active during the War. I was in the Army, too. I was a driver for a Brigadier, I was his chauffeur. I was based out at Lincolnshire, in Digby, at the Canadian Air Force Station. After the War, my husband and I both came back to Hereford. My husband worked at Thorn Lightings, in Hereford, for 21 years.

It's amazing the people you meet. Since coming to the hospice, I've met a few people from Holme Lacy, three of them, in fact. They're people who I've known over the years. It's funny how you meet people after all these years. There was a man I met four years ago, Bill, who used to live in Holme Lacy. I knew him for two days at the hospice but he passed away very quickly. He wasn't very well, really. But I had two good mornings with him, nattering away about old times.

I've got osteoporosis in my bones and I've got cancer in my stomach too. The osteoporosis has been there for quite a few years, but the cancer has only been with me for six months or so. They won't operate because of my age. The surgeon told me I might not heal properly. She persuaded me not to have anything done and I've gone a few months since and it's not too bad. My bones are painful, they are, very painful. If I have to walk, it hurts. If it wasn't for the osteoporosis I could walk about a bit better, which I'd like. But the cancer hasn't been too bad, it's been behaving itself.

I've had quite a bit of bad health myself but I keep getting through it. I was in hospital for all kinds of other things when they discovered the cancer.

They told me six months ago. I can't do anything about it. What can you do? You've got to have a sense of humour about it. It's no good going under. I'm still going along alright. I don't feel too bad in myself. It's no good sitting around doing nothing.

When I'm at home, I do a bit of knitting. I can't do as much as I used to. My hands get a bit numb and my arms won't let me do it. But I do knitting for my daughter, who lives in Canada. I make the socks for her table sales and things like that.

My children are one of the greatest blessings in my life. I've got six in all, including twins who you can't tell apart. There's grandchildren, too, but there's too many to remember. I think there's 10 of them. And then there's the great-grandchildren too. I love seeing them. I've got good children, really. They look after me and take me out a lot. One of them took me out yesterday for a few hours, but these days I'd rather stay home and relax instead.

I'd heard about the hospice from my friends and I'm glad I did because I do enjoying coming here. The staff are marvellous, you can't fault them. And their meals are beautiful, I have dinner here. It's lovely.

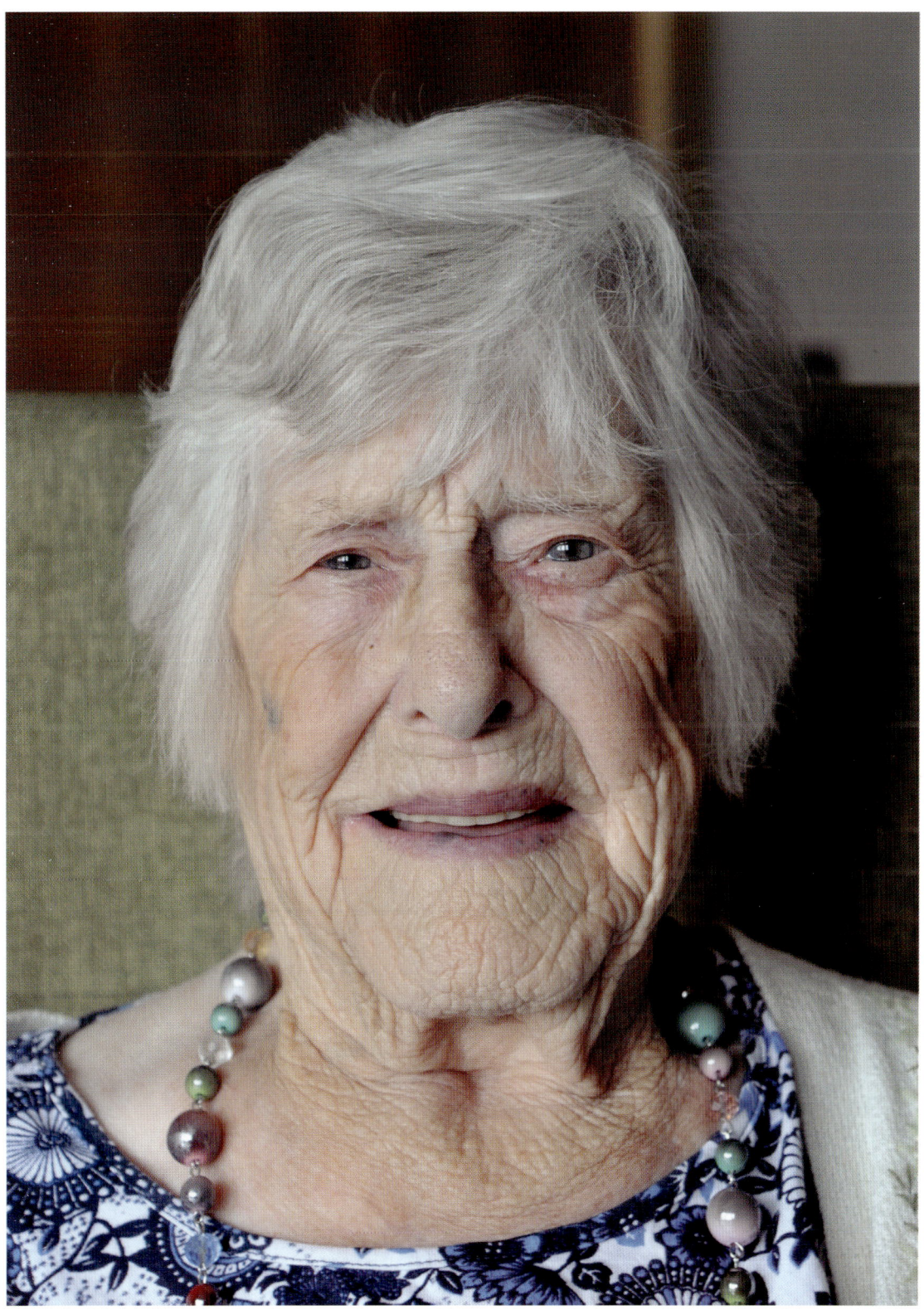

Fiona Barrett, 78 Clungunford

I came to the hospice on Tuesday last week. I had been at home before that.

I have got MND, which is a progressive illness. I haven't spoken for two or three years, I communicate by typing words on an iPad. It takes me a long time and writing a single sentence can take several minutes. It is not easy.

I have not eaten for 20 months. I am fed through a tube.

I lived for a long time in London, then I moved to Hereford.

I am an artist and spent most of my time working as a sculptress. After completing my degree at university, I became an artist. I also did my post-graduate studies at the Courtauld Institute of Art, in London. It was part of the University of London. After that, I was a teacher and worked at art colleges as well as doing my own work full-time. I specialised in fairly modern art. I love art from the late 19th century.

Most of my painting was for my own enjoyment. I also travelled a lot. I loved walking holidays and going to places where there were no roads but lots of peace. I found it very inspirational. I went to the Himalayas on six occasions and I climbed a little, too. I would go on very steep hills, but nothing that involved ropes.

It tires me to talk for a long time. After 15 minutes my energy goes and today has been a very chaotic day. I'd like to say a few things about the people at St Michael's.

The staff at St Michael's are remarkable. They are the opposite of cruel, the opposite of the cruelty of Isis. Not only that, they have never been impatient. They are so kind.

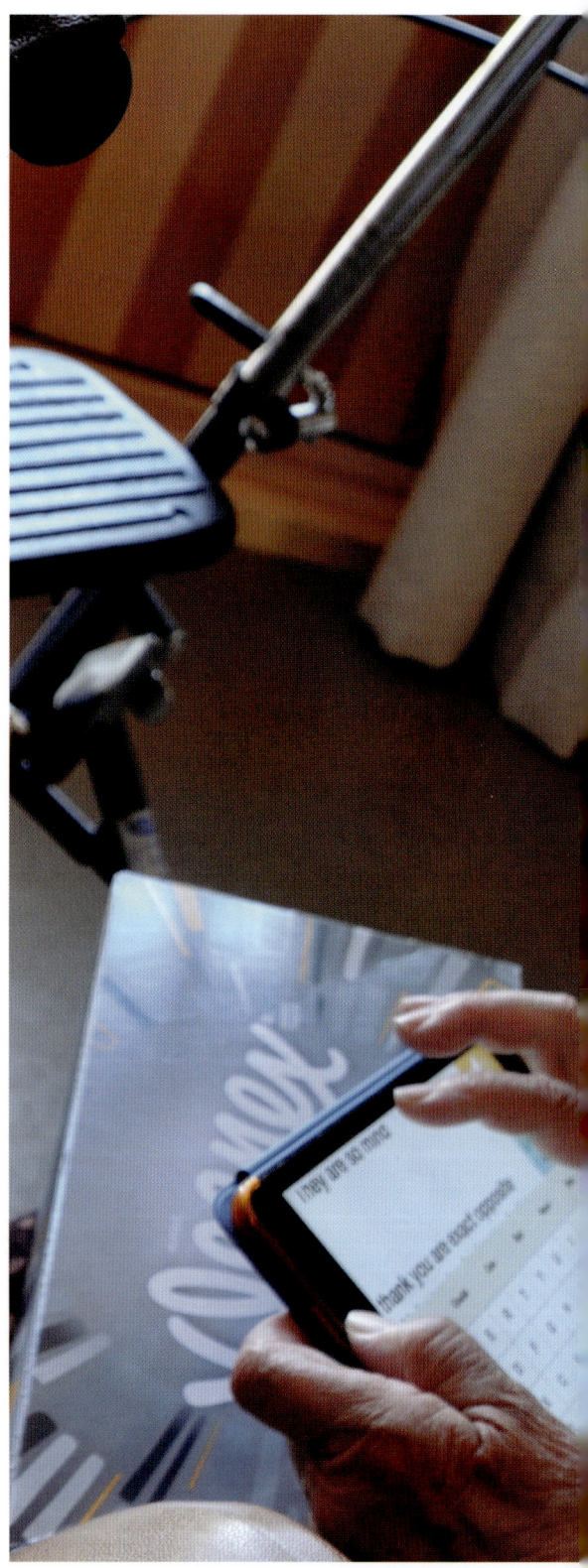

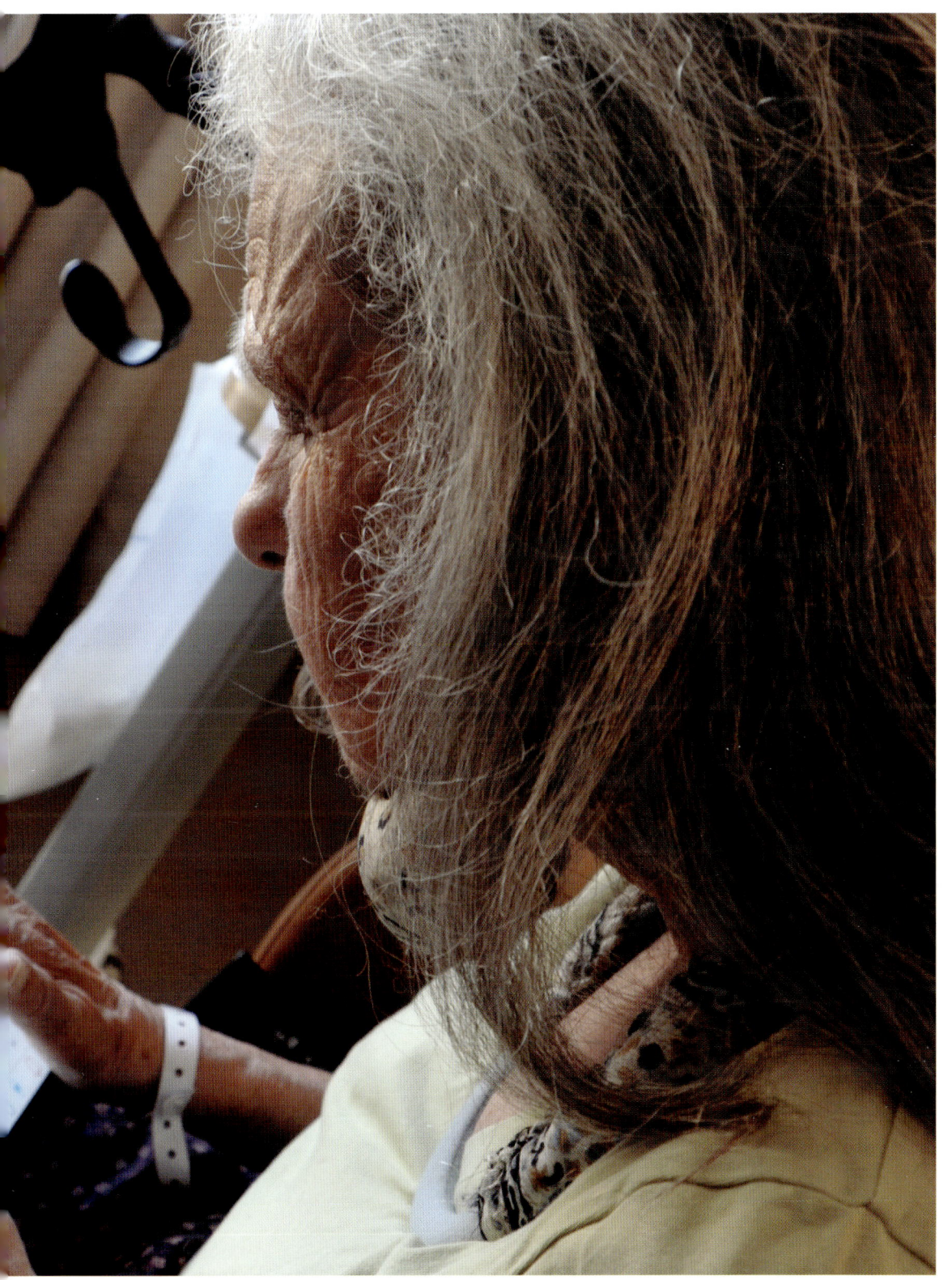

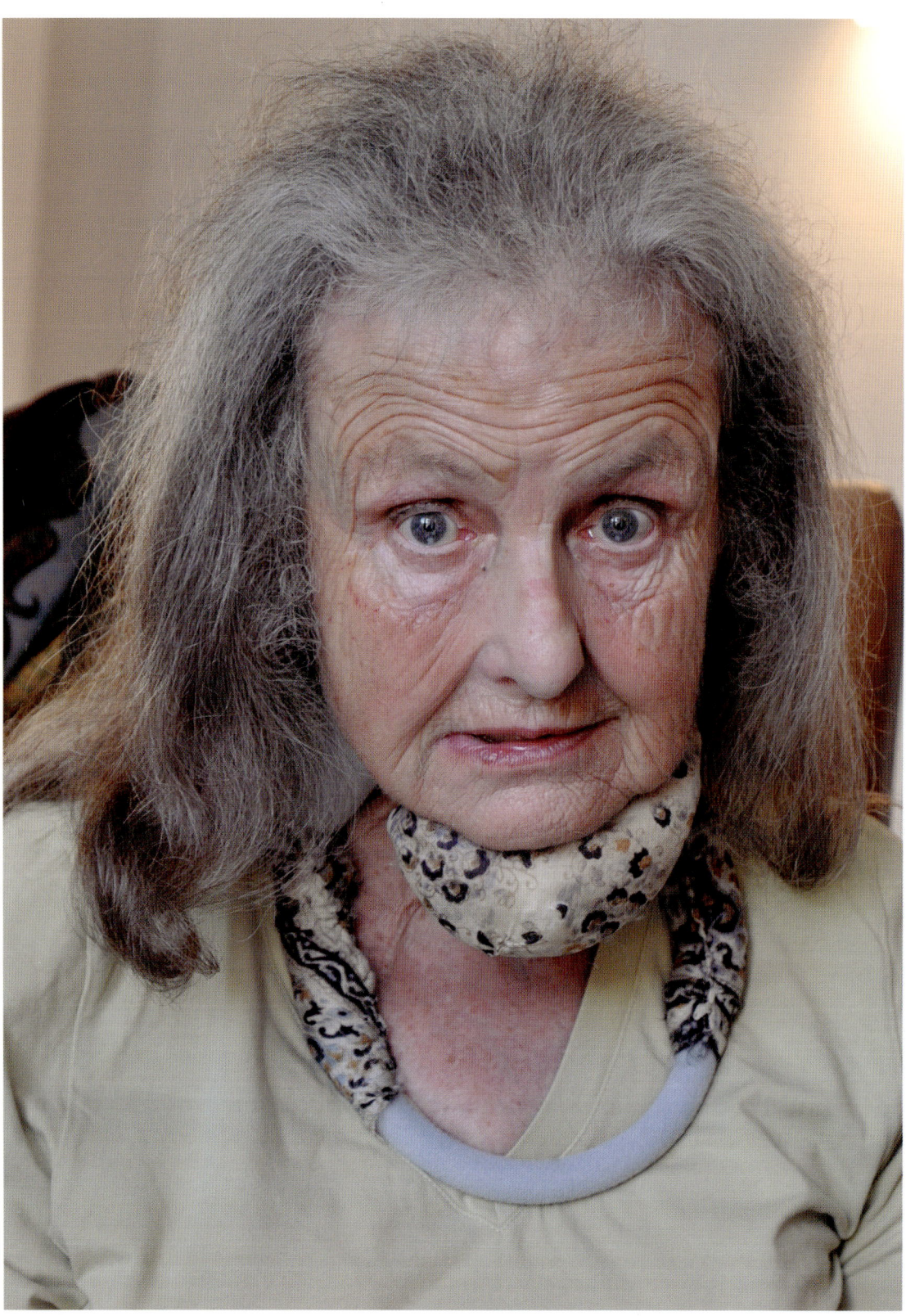

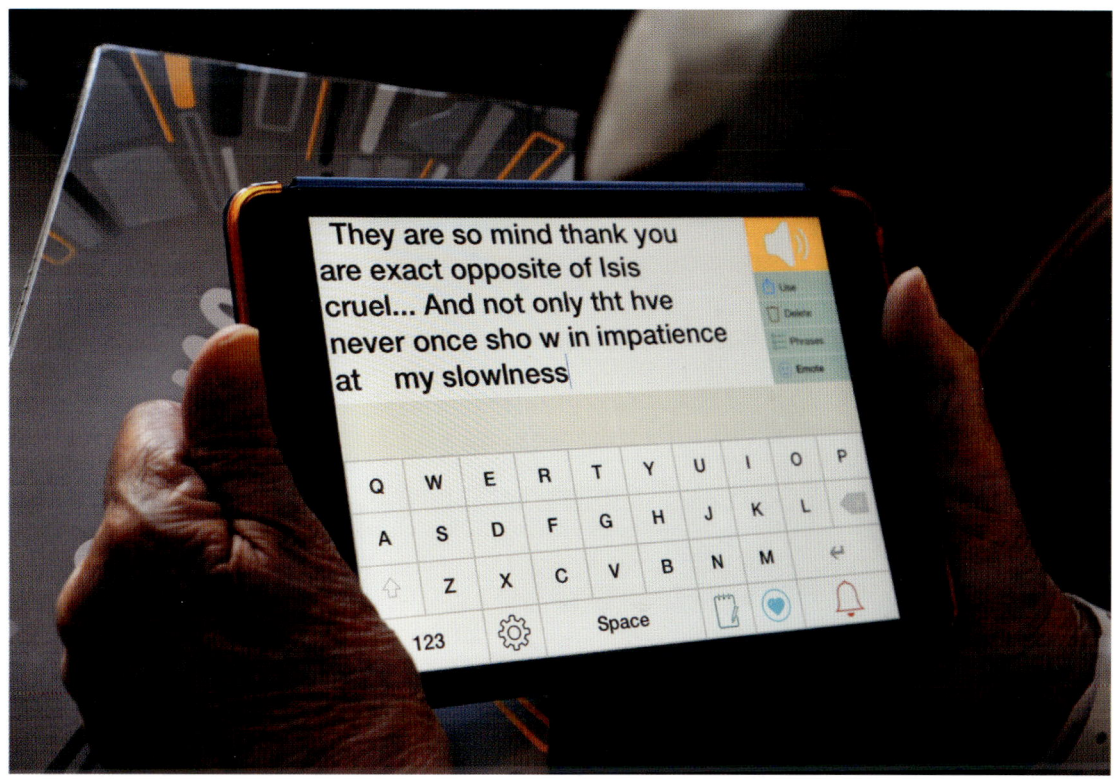

'I have got MND, which is a progressive illness. I haven't spoken for two or three years, I communicate by typing words on an iPad. It takes me a long time and writing a single sentence can take several minutes. It is not easy.'

John Hollis, 72
Llangarron

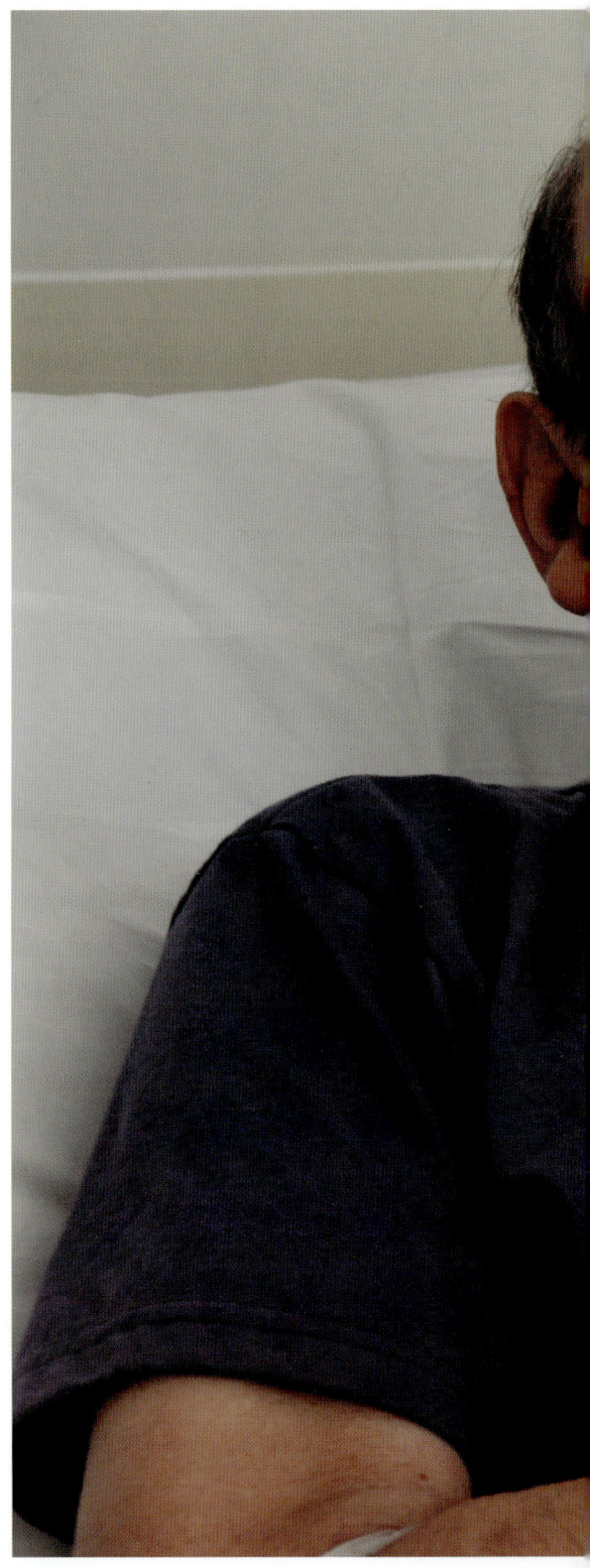

'm from Birmingham, from Tyseley and Lea Village, to be precise. I was brought up in East Birmingham.

We moved to Northamptonshire first and lived there for about 10 years. After that, we moved to Herefordshire. We've spent 40 something years in Herefordshire, the whole family are more or less over here.

I've got five kids and loads of grandchildren. I can count them still, but it will take me a while. My head's a bit fuzzy today. I can't remember numbers so well. I've been like that for a little while, not great. Any questions with sums or numbers take me a little while.

I came in about 12 or 13 days ago. I'd been at home before that but ill for a while.

Since coming in here, they've found out what's wrong and started to put me back on track. The difference in my health has been amazing, I must admit.

To be honest, I've been ill for much, much longer.

I've been poorly for about 10 years. I've had miloma cancer, off and on, and I haven't been able to work since it came.

But things came to a head recently. Nobody was able to sort things out but since I've come in here, things have really picked up.

I came in about 13 days ago. At that point, I didn't even know what day it was or where I was. It was terrible. I'd never had nothing like it before, I'd never been that ill. It felt really real. It was frightening. But within three days of coming in here, I was back on my feet.

They've been amazing here; really, really, really amazing. The care has been unbelievable. Nothing is too much trouble. To get from where I was to

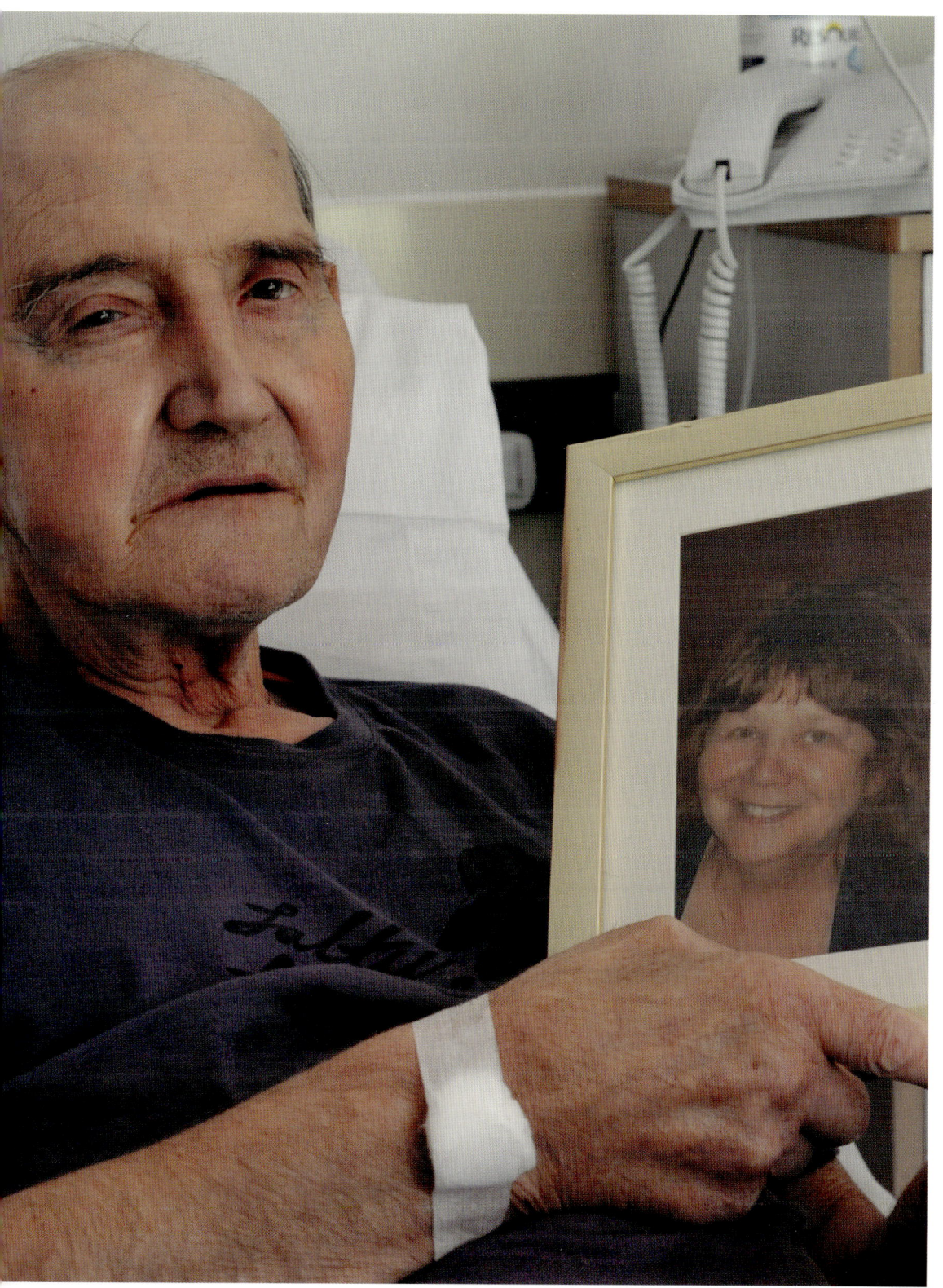

where I am now in three days has been incredible. I can't believe it. I really thought that was it, you know. I thought I was gone.

I've always suffered with a weak chest, that's been going on for a long time. I've had pneumonia a couple of times and things like that. But until now, it hadn't come up to anything.

Things were getting worse and worse but I didn't want to come to the hospice or hospital. I wanted to soldier on.

My daughters begged me to come in but I just didn't want to do it. I didn't think I'd come out if I came in. But they begged me to come in and get some help.

When I came in, I thought that would be it. Things had been getting worse all the time and I didn't know where I was or what time of day it was.

It wasn't so much pain, it was more confusion.

I'd never been like that before. I thought I was gone. I'd never had anything like that in my life. It was frightening.

Since coming in, I've been so quick in getting better. I can't understand how I could have been that ill and then three days later I'm walking around.

Over the years, I've learned how to cope with being ill.

When the cancer was first diagnosed, 10 years ago, I had stem cell replacement. That was the first big thing. It had a positive effect but it took ages to make a difference. It really was a slow process. My wife kept me going for the first seven years of that, but she passed away three years ago.

Her name was Sheila and I keep her photograph with me. She was my strength.

Since my wife went, my children have been my strength. They have been great, really devotional. I don't know what I'd have done without them.

At first it was Sheila but in the past three years it's been the kids. It couldn't have been better with my family. I'm a lucky man and I know it.

The illness got to a point where it was just easier to lie back and let it roll over the top of me. I couldn't do anything about it. I couldn't function. I was just getting worse. I couldn't remember telephone numbers, which was one of the most frightening things.

My daughter was living next door, which was handy. I built a house for my mum and dad, years ago, but they both got ill over the years and passed away during the 10 years that they were there. Then when I got ill, my daughter moved in next door so that she could look after me. She's one of five, as I said. I've got two daughters and three boys and my daughters take it in turns to look after me.

Living at home was a battle and everything changed when my wife died. I used to enjoy fishing and a wide variety of things, mostly sports. But my enjoyment seemed to stop after my wife died. Before that, I'd enjoy working outside on the fences and with the sheep on our land. But I

> '**My wife kept me going for the first seven years of that, but she passed away three years ago. Her name was Sheila and I keep her photograph with me.**'

slowly stopped wanting to do things after Sheila died. I sort of gave up a little bit. There wasn't any motivation.

I could still see what the kids were doing for me, I wasn't entirely selfish.

It was the opposite, to be honest, I was very grateful for what they were doing. But I was very low. I just thought: 'Why am I bothering?' That's how I felt after Sheila passed. I wasn't really poorly after Sheila went but I wasn't well.

I was mobile up to a point but slowly I lost that. Initially, I did my own shopping and cooked myself a bit of dinner but over time, I stopped wanting to do it. It might seem like a tale of misery but that's the way it was. After Sheila went, I couldn't help changing.

But being in the hospice has given me a big kick up the backside. I think I came to a bridge when I came in here. Before, I couldn't see what I was doing and I couldn't carry on.

I couldn't carry on putting my kids through what they've been through. So somewhere a decision had to be made. And I've decided to make the best of things from now on.

The point before I came here was the lowest point of my life.

I can trace it all back to Sheila.

After Sheila's death, I got more and more down. Then, when they brought me in here, I realised I had two choices. I could either carry on or not.

It wasn't fair to keep going with things the way they were, it wasn't fair on anybody. What the kids were doing to look after me was unbelievably unselfish.

They were spending more and more time with me, even though they still had their own families to run.

I got to the point where I was ready for the worst. I'd been getting ready for that since losing Sheila, really. I just couldn't see any way out. That was over that period of three years. That's when it really took a turn.

We'd been married for 49 years and nothing can replace that. There's no replacement. But then again there's no replacement for the kids, either.

They've dedicated their lives to me for the last three years even though they have families of their own. From their perspective, it's been total dedication.

It's more than anybody should ask.

When all this started, we had a big long chat about it. I'd got some experience of being ill, from the last time when I had the miloma. I knew it was going to be rough.

'. . . being in the hospice has given me a big kick up the backside. Before, I couldn't see what I was doing and I couldn't carry on.'

I told them I didn't want to put them through it because it would be too long and too hard.

But they wouldn't have it any other way. They haven't complained about it, never once.

Funny things come out of people, I think, at funny times and this has brought out the best of them.

I often think about how much they've done for me.

I think that people might be able to keep things going for a week or a fortnight or a month; but to do things for month after month after month and year after year, it's hard.

And at the back of your mind, you know you're not going to get better. There's no cure. Even after the stem cell replacement, I knew it would come back. You just have to deal with it as best as you can.

Now that I'm in the hospice, at least three or four of the kids come in every day. It's incredible. It makes me feel very humble. I think to myself: 'I couldn't do it, not spend that amount of time'.

Being in the hospice makes a big difference because the staff here are totally expert.

They seem to know what's coming next. I've had a lot to do with hospitals in the last few years but I would never have believed that this is how things could be. The level of care is incredible compared to what I've been through.

I know it's not always like this. When it is, it's spectacular.

Being here makes me wonder about why I've drifted. It's shocked me, being here. I've been getting better. I know things will never be the same again and I've got the feeling that I shouldn't really be here, that my time should have been up. That's how I feel, especially since the past few days.

I'll tell you a little bit about how I felt when I came in.

I thought I was going down, that it was over. I didn't have fear when I thought I was going to go. I've built up to that, slowly.

I think the fear of dying disappears, to be honest. I don't know about the end. You just think you won't wake up the next day.

But that's changed now. The experience here has been really good. I can't describe to you how good I feel.

I'd worked myself up to think 'the time has come now, that's it'. I slowly got used to the idea. And then you wake up the next day and you don't feel too bad. And then again the next day, you feel a little better. It's remarkable. It's amazing.

When you're in the hospice, you have a lot of time. There's time to look back over your life.

When I was working, I'd do anything that involved working outdoors. I was a builder, a plasterer, mostly. It would mostly be travelling about to Birmingham and Worcester to construction sites.

The older I got, the easier the building work got, funnily enough, because I'd learned the shortcuts.

When Shelia became ill, she quickly deteriorated. She had three months; it wasn't long, but it was long enough.

She nearly had a course of chemotherapy but that would have been totally the wrong thing for her.

We found that out afterwards. She'd got a little known illness and the chemotherapy wouldn't have worked, it would have been a waste of time. I'll always be grateful that we didn't go down that road.

> 'I'm looking forward to going home. I've got to do it sometime. I don't worry about anything now, really. There's nothing that can hurt me any more.'

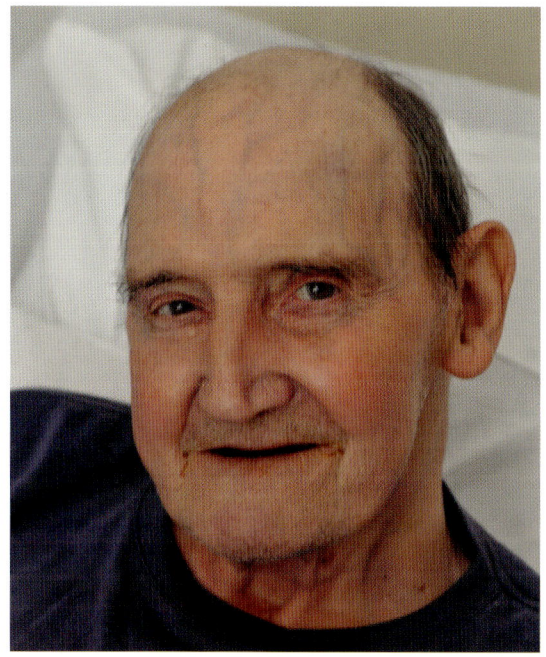

But now, I'm looking forward to going home. I've got to do it sometime.

I don't worry about anything now, really. There's nothing that can hurt me any more.

I mean, I've never had much money or anything like that but we've always managed. I always found plenty of work, as much as I ever needed.

I have no fears about going home now. Coming here woke me up.

I tell you what: somebody came from somewhere to help me, that's for sure, because I didn't know where to go, at all.

This crew here, honestly, they have been unbelievable, all of them, every single one.

Now, I think: 'What can happen?' Nothing can happen. I'm alright'.

I think about the happy times. When I was first ill and at home with my wife, I enjoyed it.

It seems funny, but having all that time at home, even though I was ill, was a blessing.

I'd never had any time off from work before. I'd never had any time off, in fact. I used to wake up in the morning and think 'great, I haven't got to go to work'.

Me and Sheila were both at home together and I enjoyed it. We used to laugh and joke and I'd get under her feet, as usual.

I was never one for the TV, but I used to like music.

We had a smallholding, not that we could make any money from it. We used to have sheep on the land and I'd spend my time mending fences. There was always something to do. My wife would always find me something to do.

I think I'm lucky. It's been very hard, but hopefully we're through the worst now.

For the kids' sake, I hope things get better. They deserve a break. They are brilliant. They are really good.

The big difference between being at the hospice and being somewhere else is that the people here care. They truly care. You can tell the difference.

I've never had that much to complain about at hospitals.

When I was at Hereford Hospital, the people there were brilliant.

I've been in and out of there for 10 years and they've told me what's going to happen next and not tried to hide. They've given it me straight. So when things have happened, they've not been that much of a surprise. I've known the cancer would come back, they've always made that clear.

Knowing what's happening has always helped me to deal with things much better.

They also give you hope.

Until a week ago, I wasn't particularly bothered about going home. I was quite willing to just stop and see what happens, which isn't like me.

But that was because I was so down and also because my wife had died, that's the only reason I thought about giving up.

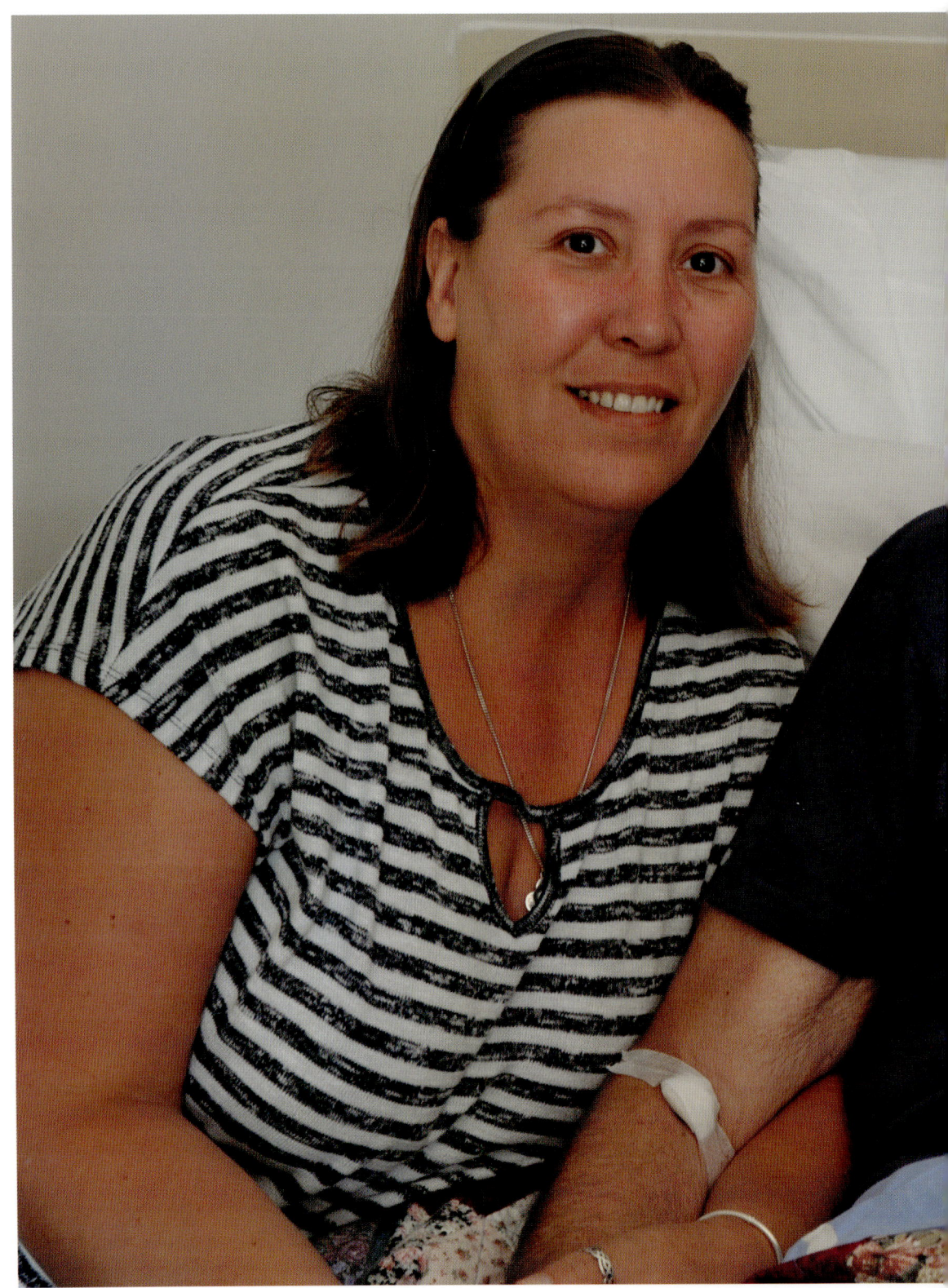

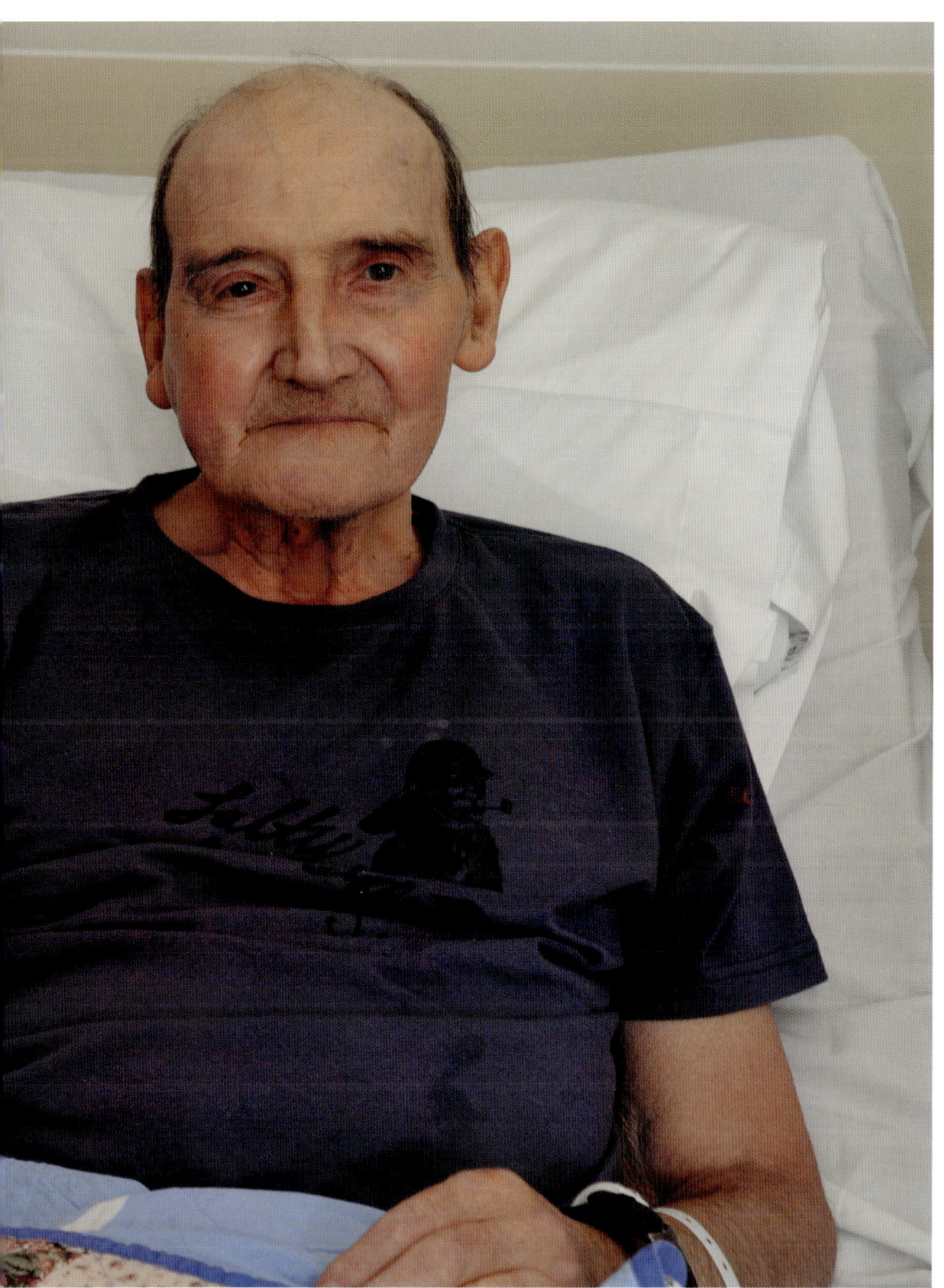

Marian and Dennis Bennett, both 80
Newton Farm, Hereford

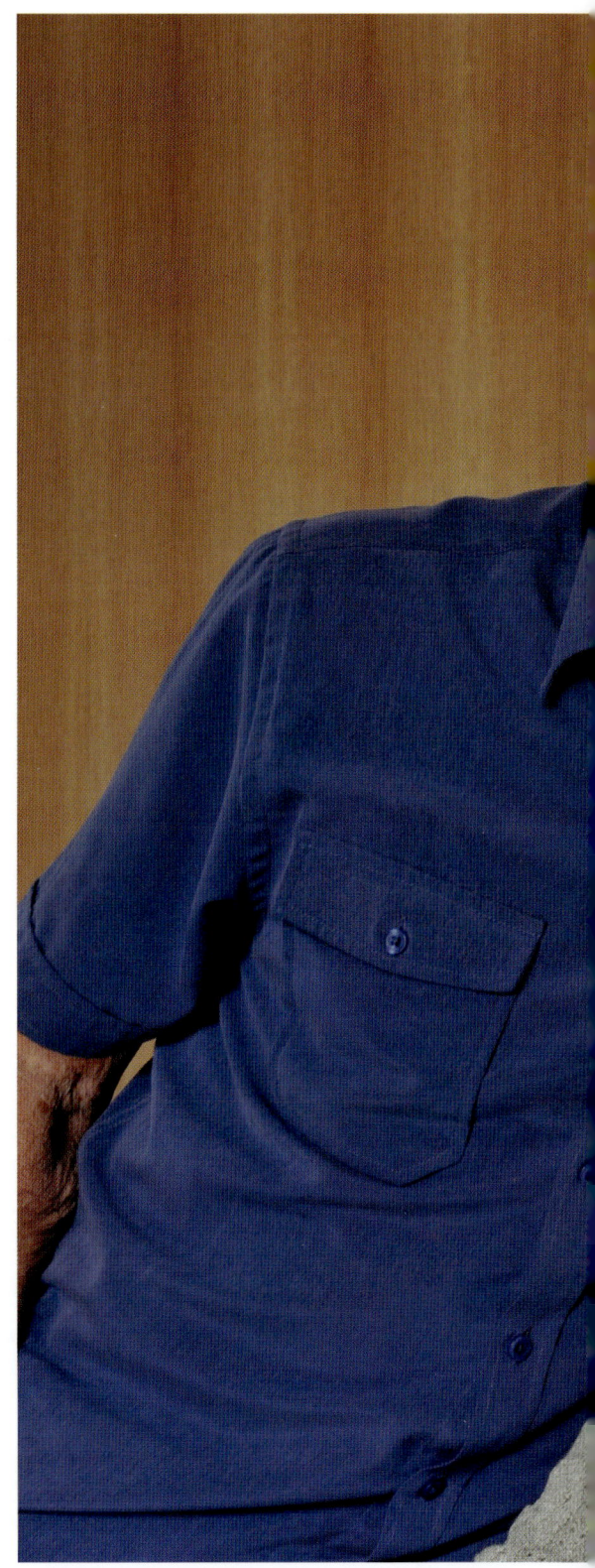

Marian: "I came here 12 days ago and I hope to go home later today. Things are looking good. I was very poorly when I was admitted. At that point, I was being sick every day. The sickness had gone on for eight or nine weeks, it was terrible.

A nurse from the hospice, called Becky, used to come and visit us. We'd speak to her about what was going on. We gradually started to realise that the tablets being prescribed by the doctor weren't working and Becky told us we needed to do something. She said: 'This can't go on'. She talked to us and said she would see about us coming into the hospice."

Dennis: "The great myth about the hospice is that it's the place where you go to die. It's not. It might have been years ago, but that's not the case anymore.

"People used to come in and gradually pass away. But that's all changed now. They've got a brand new building and it's terrific. The rooms are lovely, the showers are lovely, it's all first class. Actually, it's unbelievable. We came in and Marian started her treatment straight away. Touch wood, everything has improved every day since she's been here. We are 12 days in and should be going home. I know that the word 'hospice' makes people feel a bit worried. But now that we've been here, we know better."

Marian: "I know I have cancer but we were

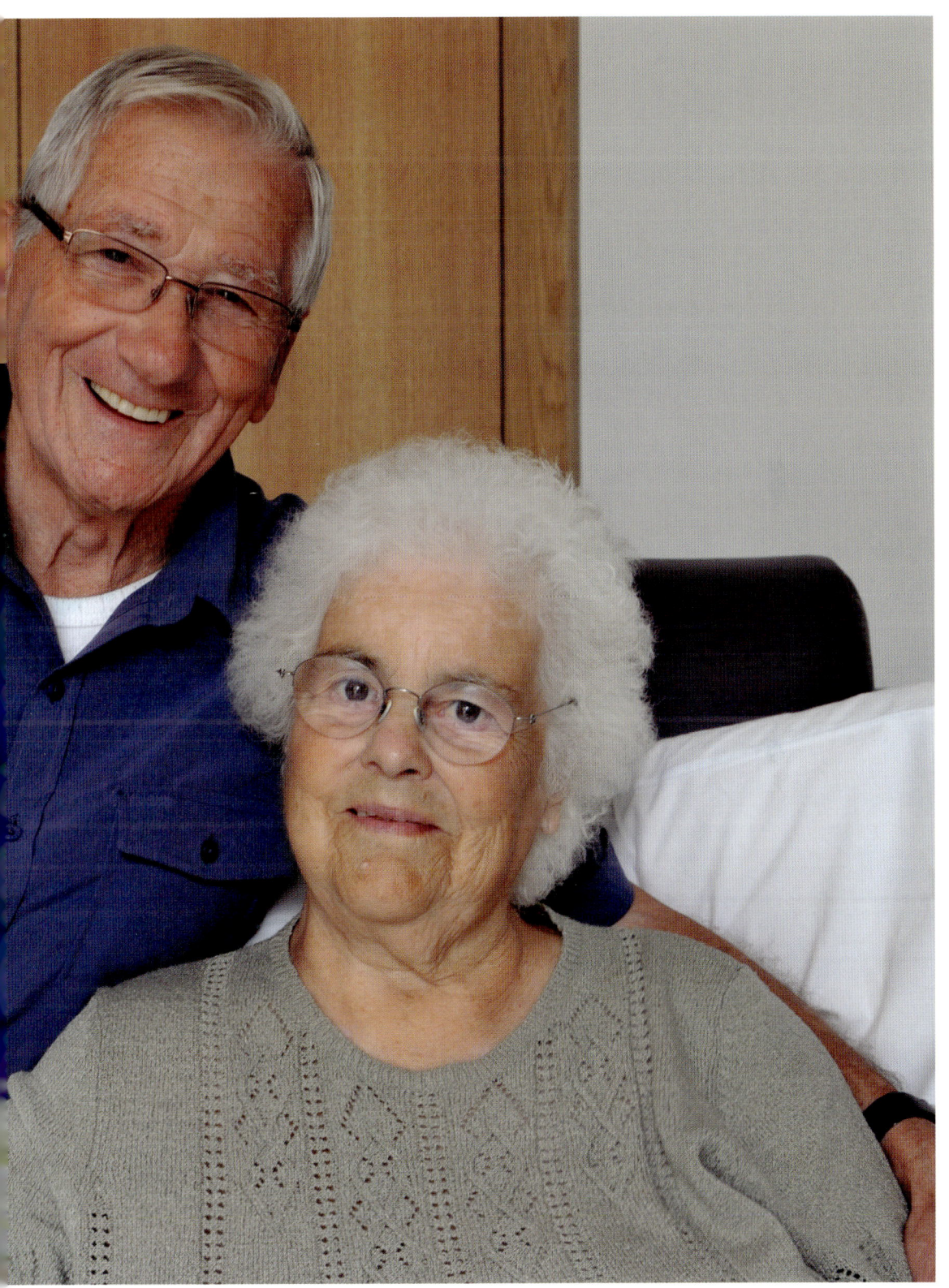

told that I could come here to get better, you know. They told us that. The idea of a hospice has changed a lot. These days, you get treatment for what you've got and for the pain that you are in. They help to make you better.

"Since I've been here, they've helped to get me off the tablets and back on my feet. They've cut down my tablets by half and I'm a lot, lot, lot better. The atmosphere is very relaxed and that helps to put people at ease. It's very casual and there's no rushing about. There's no: 'Here's your dinner, eat this'. There are no Sergeant Majors. They treat the patients like friends. They come in and ask you each day what you want for your meal. Even Dennis can order a meal."

Dennis: "When people get ill, the focus is naturally on the patient. And that's the way it should be. But there's also additional stresses and strains for the carer. And the hospice understands that. They help me as well as Marian."

Marian: "They always ask if Dennis is alright. They help to give the carer a rest, a break. It's not just about the person who's ill. It's also about the person who looks after them as well."

Dennis: "Before Marian came in, she was awake most of the night, rocking back and forth, feeling sick. Then once she'd been sick, the nausea and the pain would ease off a bit."

Marian: "I'd go to sleep for a bit. Then I'd be up in the morning and I'd stay downstairs for a bit. But pretty soon I'd have to go back to bed.

"I came into the hospice and they put me on injections and then on a machine, an anti-sickness machine. I was bad the first day. But then my body started to respond. I've been okay since the first day.

"I get up at breakfast time, there's no rush. It's not up at 7am on the dot. I can get up and have breakfast at 8am or 8.30am or whenever I wake up. The nurses are coming in and out all the time asking me: 'Are you alright?' There's lots of space, there's a TV, there's a garden outside my window."

Dennis: "They really try and look after people. You don't have to pay for your own TV or telephone. They just tell you not to call Australia or New Zealand, because that would cost too much!"

Marian: "Dennis comes first thing in the morning and goes home about 4pm to have a bit of tea and a break. He can order meals whenever he likes while he's here.

"The biggest thing the hospice has done is helped to cure the sickness. The sickness was worse than the pain. I had constant nausea. I've got other problems. I was diagnosed as having cancer last October. Instead of going for chemotherapy, I have it in tablet form. I had a CT scan last Thursday and we're just waiting for the result of that.

"Another thing about the hospice is that it's very positive. They just get on with things and do it. I am going home with a lot less tablets to when I came in. I used to be on diabetes tablets, but I'm

> '**You don't have to pay for your own TV or telephone. They just tell you not to call Australia or New Zealand, because that would cost too much!'**

off those completely."

Dennis: "She used to be on so many pills in the morning and in the afternoon. It would be 17 or 18 tablets a day by the time she'd taken them all. Now it's halved."

Marian: "The hospice has also taken away the strain. We used to have a lot to do. Dennis did the lot, to be honest. He would clean the house, do the shopping and take care of me; everything. He also helped me manage with being sick. When I was at home, I spent about eight or nine weeks walking around with a sick bowl, in case I vomited. I would be sick everywhere. I'd have an appointment with the Macmillan nurses or at the doctor's surgery and I'd just be sick in the car. Even if I was waiting in the surgery or at Macmillan, I'd have to have a bowl because I could be sick at any moment. It was uncontrollable.

"Now that's calmed down. I get some rest each night and Dennis can get a sleep when he goes home. I'm not waking him all the time, the way I was. I feel 1,000 times better. When I was sick, I lost weight and it took it out of me. But now I just sit down and I enjoy a meal. I know my meals are still small, but they're nice.

"When I was ill, I'd just eat mashed potato because I couldn't manage any meat. For a while, I thought it was meat that was making me ill. I couldn't eat eggs, either. But I've been able to eat everything again since I came here.

"Before, I couldn't taste my food. But that's all changed. I had a nice sandwich the other day, an egg mayonnaise sandwich. It was the best one I've had in my life. It was lovely."

Dennis: "The hospice has been good for all of us. It's accommodated our family, as well as Marian and I. We live on the Newton Farm Estate, by Hereford, and we've been married for 57 years. We've got two boys, two girls and we've got four grandchildren; three girls and a boy. We've got five great grandchildren too. The granddaughters and great grandkiddies come here to see Marian and it's lovely. They can run around or go outside.

"I remember years ago, when my own mum was in hospital. In those days, children weren't allowed to go in to the ward to see their parents. I remember once, I went up to the end of the corridor and one of the sisters saw me. She was feeling kind and decided to let me on the ward. She pointed to where my mum was and said: 'Get up there, go on lad, be quick'. And I ran up there to see my mother and give her a hug and a kiss then I came back. But they never allowed children other than that. But here, it's totally different. There's an open door. Years ago the kiddies couldn't go in. These days, all the little kiddies are walking around and they can go out and play outside, it's lovely."

'There's an open door. Years ago the kiddies couldn't go in. These days, all the little kiddies are walking around and they can go out and play outside, it's lovely."

Marian: "The family can come and relax. My two daughters both had the same week off, last week. Of course, when they booked their holiday, they didn't know I would be here. They were coming in from 10am in the morning and they'd sit all day with me and go for walks and things. It's been lovely. And being in that sort of environment also makes me feel better. We have the family here and they sit here laughing. The fun you can have is amazing. We have so much fun. Dennis tries to help me into bed and then he'll joke with me and give me a smack and tell me to hurry up. He's a laugher and a joker. Anyone outside would be thinking 'what's the matter with them'. But that's the way the place is. People don't come in with a long face or anything. The staff are terrific. They are bright in the morning and afternoon. They all call me 'love, dear, darling', it's wonderful. They remember my name, too. They don't forget me. It's great."

Dennis: "The staff have been brilliant, brilliant, they have. If Marian has had to call them in at night time, she's said: 'I'm sorry to disturb you'. But they tell her not to worry. They say: 'That's what we're here for, that's our job, you call us any time of day or night'. We're not on our best behaviour, we can just be ourselves. The staff are all on first name terms, they treat us like friends. They were friendly with us from the beginning. They have got time for us."

Marian: "When it's time to take my tablets, they explain what I'm having and why I'm having it. They take away the anxiety of being ill. They're not rushing in and doing things too quickly. They come along and they say: 'Right, hang on Marian,

I've just got to go and get something, I'll be back'. They're good communicators. They treat the patients with a lot of love and respect and care. It's relaxed from day one.

"We've lived a long life and it's nice that people care. When I was much younger, I had my children and then stayed at home to look after them. Then I went out on the land, on the farms, to work. I'd take the kiddies with me. Once they'd grown up and could look after themselves, I went to work at Sun Valley, the chicken factory. Dennis used to work at Wiggins as well as Sun Valley. Then he went to Bulmers."

Dennis: "Being in the hospice has given us time to reflect. We're looking forward to our birthdays; mine is in October and Marian's is in March.

"We've spent our lives together. We met at Wormelow Dancehall. I think we met on the bus. We were coming back from Wormelow into Hereford and I was sitting down. Marian was standing up and I said: 'Do you want a seat, dear?' She said 'yes'. So I slapped my lap and said: 'Come and sit on my lap, then'. We've been making each other laugh ever since."

Marian: "He was always a bit of a charmer. I think when we met he was on leave from the army, he had just been demobbed. He had done his National Service. He'd been in the army in 1955 and came out in '57 after two years' National Service. He served in Kenya, in Nairobi. Then he went back up the Suez Canal and was

> 'People don't come in with a long face or anything. The staff are terrific. They are bright in the morning and afternoon. It's wonderful.'

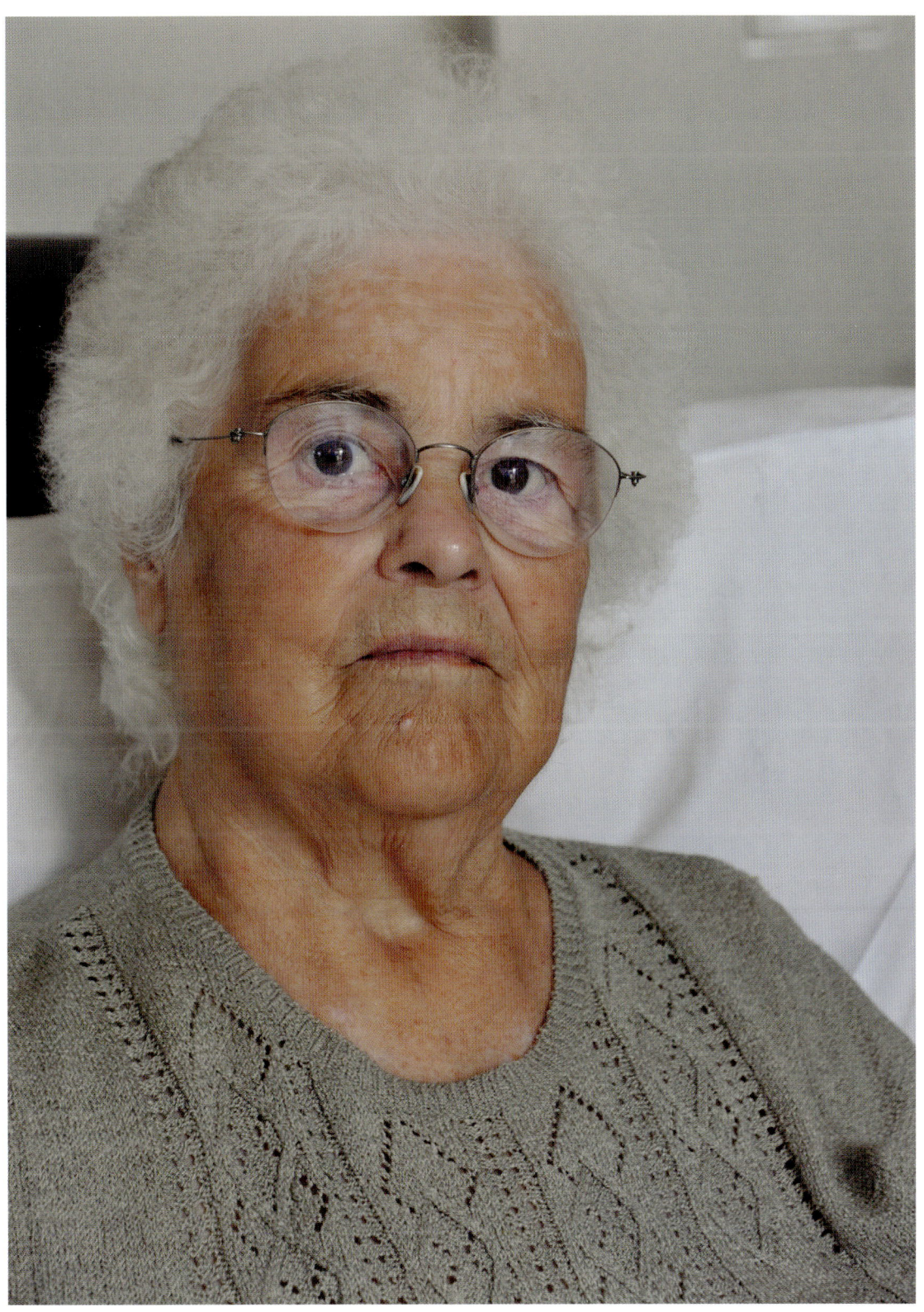

in Bahrain. Then it was back to Nairobi before coming home.

"I still remember the days when we were courting. Dennis used to go out at dinner time and have a few beers and on Saturday it would be dance night. I'd like to go to the pictures on a Saturday and then Dennis and I would go to meet my mum and dad and we'd all have a drink towards the end of the evening.

"We were courting for two years before we got married. We got married in Hereford, in St Martin's Church. We didn't have a honeymoon because Dennis had to go back to work on the Monday."

Dennis: "We had a holiday later. I think the first holiday was Tenby. We used to go there quite a bit. We had a caravan there and then we had the kids. We upgraded to our own tent, then we had a trailer tent, then we upped a little bit more to a caravan.

"We still love to travel now, when we can. Our granddaughter buys us a holiday for a Christmas present. We used to go to a place called Dawlish Warren, down in Devon. The holidays are lovely because we don't want any presents, we don't want the kids or grandkids to waste their money."

Marian: "It was only by chance that I found out I was ill. I had a very bad cold. I was coughing and coughing and I rubbed all down my side. I was aching. I felt down my side and felt something, a lump. I thought: 'What's that?' So I went straight to the doctor. I told Dennis and the kids first. We went to the doctor and it all went from there.

"We were together when the doctor told us. The doctor told us he'd have it investigated and then we went to Macmillan for the biopsy. The cancer was in the breast, stomach and groin. They told us there wouldn't be any operations but they'd put me on tablets, instead of chemotherapy. Touch wood, it's started to get better. The lump is going down and we're getting good results. Now we're waiting to hear about the CT scan.

"Having the support of the hospice and the love of my family makes a difference. I was bad for such a long time but things are getting better. From nowhere, it's all getting better. I was being sick all the time, it was pumping out, it was like a tap being turned on. Whenever I ate, it came out. I had potatoes one day and they tasted of vinegar. I thought the potatoes were bad but everyone told me they were fine, it was me. Now, since I've been in the hospice, they've sorted all that out. I can eat again without being sick.

"It's been good to come to the hospice but I'm looking forward to going home. I'm looking forward to being in my own bed. I want to have a good night's sleep back home. When I get out, Dennis will be back to his allotment and we'll be back to normal. We can't wait."

Dennis: "All we want is to get her home. They are nice here, don't get me wrong. But there's no place like home."

"All we want is to get her home. They are nice here, don't get me wrong. But there's no place like home."

Christine Wilson, 67 Hereford

I hope you don't mind if I don't have my photograph taken. I'm happy to talk about St Michael's, it's certainly been enormously helpful in my case.

But I'm not the sort of person who's comfortable with their photograph being taken, so I'll skip on that and tell you my story, instead, if that's okay. I'll have to drink while I'm talking to you because the drugs make my mouth very dry.

I'm originally from Hull, but I've been in Hereford for about 17 years now. I met my girlfriend here. I'd been working abroad and I came back for a while for a break. A friend of ours introduced us and we've been together ever since. I'd been working abroad as a secretary for a large organisation in Saudi Arabia. We bought a house not long after we met, 15 or 16 years ago, and she stayed here. She's a nurse, her name's Caroline.

I left school when I was 15 and took up work as an office junior. I went to night school and did shorthand and typing and so on. I was pretty good at shorthand; I was about 140 words per minute. I had various jobs in Hull, including a job at the hospital as a medical secretary. One of the girls, Rosemary, brought an advert for secretaries, working in Saudi. She couldn't afford to go to London for the interviews, so I asked if she'd mind if I had a go. So I went down, had the interview, got the job and that was it.

Actually, I've skipped ahead. That happened more recently. If you want me to go right back to the start, I had another overseas position, which was at NATO, in Brussels. That was in 1971. I stayed there for five years. I came back and met a

girl who I became involved with, though it didn't work out too well, so I went back to NATO and did another five years.

I eventually came back properly around 1986/87 but I couldn't settle in England, so I went back abroad. I could afford lots of things but my friends could only afford to do one thing. I could go for a drink, go to the cinema or go for dinner. I'd saved up while I was at NATO. You know, you can't really compare Hull with Brussels, it's a different lifestyle altogether. When I was at NATO, we'd go to France, Germany, the Netherlands and all that sort of thing. We had a very good social life and a very good sporting life, too.

NATO was a fascinating place to work. During my first stint there, I worked for the military, as a civilian. NATO is split into two parts, with the civilian part and the military part. The political wing accounts for about three-quarters of it. I worked for the MBFR team, which stands for Mutual and Balanced Force Reductions. During my first time there, there were a lot of talks about the Warsaw Pact, in Vienna. It was a very interesting job. I was secretary to the guy who ran the team. They would present papers to the NATO Council.

I stayed there until 1976 and had hoped to go to Canada to work after that, but they closed the doors just as I was about to go. But in the meantime, I met a girl in England, and we were together for about five years. Then we broke up so I went back to NATO, in 1981 and stayed for another five years.

Sport has always been a big part of my life, as well as work. I've always done running but then I've done five-year tranches of other sports, like tennis and squash and when I reached a certain age, 50, I concentrated on the running.

I won a few championships, particularly at running. My PB for 400m would have been just below 60 seconds, which isn't very fast. I didn't do athletics for all that long. My half-mile was about two minutes 20 seconds. Squash was a big part of my life and I played for the Yorkshire second team. I was ranked about 8th in Yorkshire, it's not very high, really. But I enjoyed it. I was still playing squash when I went back to Saudi and I ended up playing for the Belgian national team, remarkably. We went to the European Championships, which were held in Munich. We had an Irish girl at number one, I was at number two, we had a Dutch girl at number three and I think we might have had a token Belgian in, as well, at number four, and then there was a French girl at number five. It was good fun. Golf was the next sport and I got into the top 10 in Yorkshire, but it was only county level, nothing special. I played steadily, a lot, for three years. After that, I spent my time running and walking and swimming.

For a long time, I was working in Bahrain and my girlfriend and I maintained a long-distance relationship. There would be phone calls and visits and so on. We finally did a civil partnership earlier this year, after all that time.

So that's how I've spent most of my life. I ought to tell you what brings me to St Michael's, too.

Three years ago I went to the doctor. I thought I'd got problems associated with old age. The first GP I saw was useless, but after that I saw a GP I really liked and immediately I was examined. She was tremendous, she really was. There was trust and she had good skills. I had a CA125 test and the results were high, so we knew straight away. Remarkably, I felt fine. But emotionally I was pretty suspicious about it. I realised what I'd got. Having been an athlete, you tend to know your body.

So I was diagnosed with ovarian cancer. When they opened me up, it wasn't ovarian; the primary was on the appendix. However, it had spread to the ovaries and fallopian tubes. So they did a hysterectomy and I had two years of chemo. They stopped that earlier this year, though, and told me that I'd gone as far as I could with it.

The hospice has helped me tremendously. I can't speak highly enough of any of the people here. They are so concerned, they all know your name, you're not just a number. They know you, straight away: all of them, within a short time. I find myself looking at their name badges, trying to keep up. Nothing is too much trouble for them, they're happy to do whatever they can. I've only been here for four days and my partner comes to visit. They are managing the pain and the progression of the disease. They're looking to keep me here for two weeks to get on top of things. They've helped me to make remarkable progress. I feel so much better than when I came in.

Before my admission, it was all over. The whole torso was in pain, abdomen … you know, it was everywhere. On a ratio of one-10, in terms of pain, I've been to 10 and we had to call out the ambulance and I had to go to hospital.

But, you know, I've dealt with it. I had chemotherapy and it was in six-week tranches. There were going to be up to 18 sessions. So after four-or-five, I rationalised that I was a quarter of the way around the track. After nine, I was halfway round. I treated it like a programme.

I'm a great believer in traditional medicine. I think it goes hand in hand with complementary. But, you know, I just get on with it. There's no bucket list. I just get on with things. My partner has been extremely supportive. I couldn't have got this far without her. She is my rock.

'There's no bucket list. I just get on with things.'

Geraldine Parker, 53
Red Hill, Hereford

My name's Geraldine Parker and I'm 53. I've been using the hospice for seven years, though only for short periods of time. I came in three days ago on this occasion and I'll be staying for another three or four days, before going home.

I've got Parkinson's Disease and the hospice helps me more than I can explain.

It's a great place to come. I really look forward to coming here. They all know me, I think I've been here longer than anyone.

I'm very poorly, as you can see from the photographs. But just because I've got physical problems doesn't mean I don't think or feel the same as anyone else. I've got just the same emotional life as the next person. I have the same needs for friendship, companionship and support.

The hospice helped me through the darkest time of my life, when my brother died. That was five years ago. He was younger than me. We got on great; we were best friends. As kids we used to fight, but we got on well. We both had families of our own but we were very close. He had Parkinson's, too. Even now, when I think about it, it makes me sad. It's as much as I can do not to cry.

The pain is still very intense. I was very fond of him. I wanted to commit suicide when he went. But they took me under their wing, they took me into their care. They've been so good, they really have brought me to life again.

When my brother went, I was convinced he was in pain. But the hospice helped me to understand that he was at peace. That made all the difference to me. It helped me to move on. They've given me

some light, they've made me happier. I was all over the place, but they've made me feel safe. I didn't want to do anything, but they helped me move on. I love all of the people here, they are very kind to me.

I'll never forget my brother, but the pain's not as hard as it was. I've learned to live with things.

I'm in touch with the hospice all the time. I come in for respite, for a week-long period, but normally

I just come here for one day a week. Coming here gives me something to look forward to. I have my own room. There are activities and the staff know my name, they're great.

Parkinson's restricts my movement. Some days my limbs are so stiff that I can't move. It takes a long time to get up in the morning because I have to stretch. I'm having an operation on my foot in October because my foot has folded over. I can't move it, so they're going to sort out that.

I've had Parkinson's for nine years now. At first, I went into denial, but now I can cope a lot better.

Before I became ill, I was a care assistant. I would go round in my car, looking after people in their own homes.

Those days have gone. I enjoyed it, but I can't drive now.

It was hard work, but you'd put a smile on the faces of the people you'd visit and cheer them all up.

It's lovely being here for respite. The rooms have got a view out of the window onto the garden. Everything's nice and green, it's wonderful to see nature and to have such a lovely view.

The hospice organises all sorts of activities. It breaks up the day. They encourage me to talk to other people because sometimes I find that hard. The staff are great. It's not easy to socialise; I'm not shy, or anything, but I am quite cautious around other people. It takes me a while to get going and get talking, but when I do I'm not too

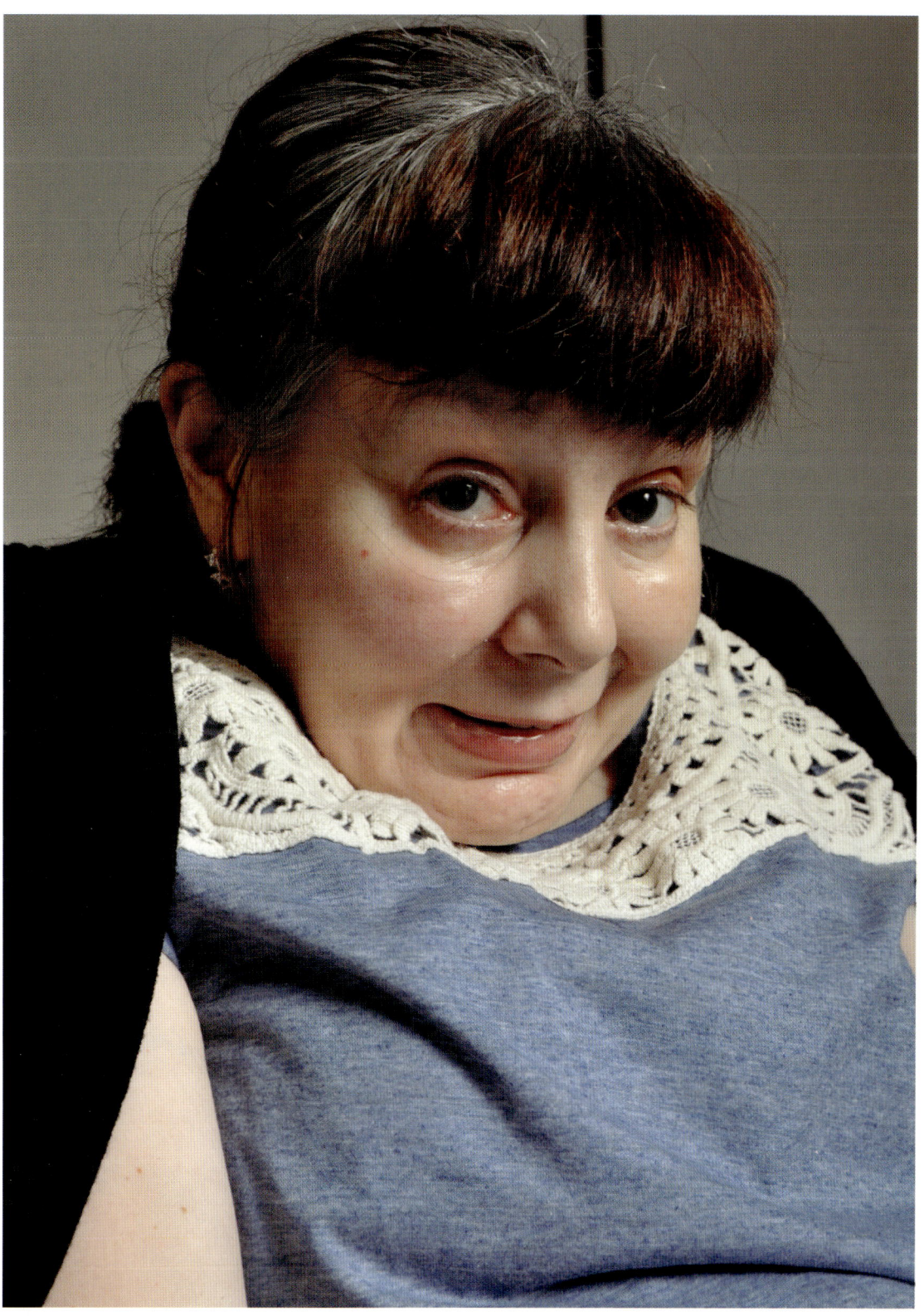

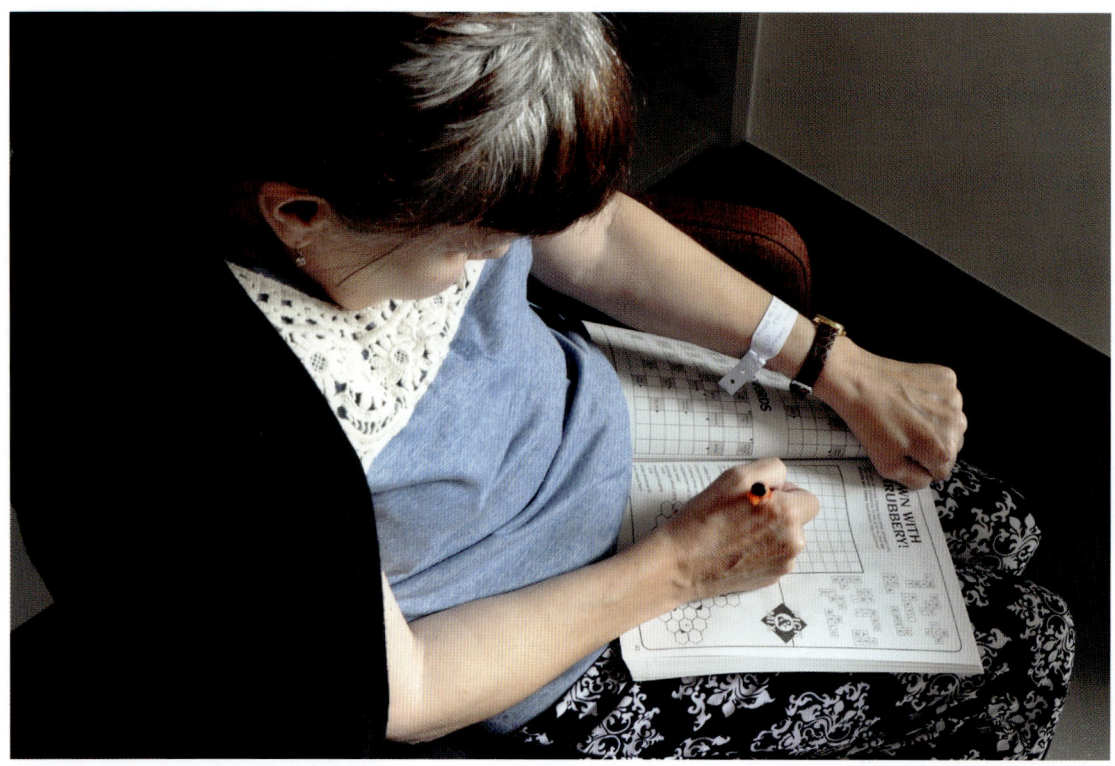

bad at all.

It's the little things that I like. When I come here, I've got a lovely soft bed. So I look forward to going to bed. My bed is much harder, at home, but the bed here is soft. I live at home with my mother. My son was there for a long time, he's 29, but he's moved out now but he still visits once or twice a week. He's got a little girl, who's three, she's called Sophia. She comes to see me and that's great. I've got lots to look forward to and enjoy.

They really help me with my Parkinson's, too. If I get a stiff neck, they can massage it and make me feel better.

You wouldn't think it, but there's a lot of laughter here. You know, they encourage me to do things, like play games in a big games room. They tell me that if other people do things I can

as well. They're supportive. They tell me: 'Come on, you've got your brain, let's use it'. It makes me positive. I use the gym, too, and that helps a lot. I go on the exercise bike and that's good for my legs, too.

The hospice understands all the things that help me and they keep me going. I love what they've done for me. They make me feel as though I've achieved something. When I have a day here, the staff cheer me up so much. I can never thank them enough.

'. . . just because I've got physical problems doesn't mean I don't think or feel the same as anyone else. I've got just the same emotional life as the next person. I have the same needs for friendship, companionship and support.'

Rhyanne Nixon, 49 Hereford

My name's Rhyanne and I have MND. I've been to St Michael's Hospice a couple of times. Once was after an operation, I was there for a month. Then, in May 2015, I was there for eight weeks.

Things had fallen apart at home, so I went there for a longer time. St Michael's helps a lot. They are very happy to have me and they try very hard. It takes a long time for people to learn about me because of my condition, but they are very, very good. They get there in the end.

I'm at a nursing home in Hereford, at Gwen Walford, but I can go back to St Michael's whenever I like. I have a free ticket.

It's difficult when you're poorly. A patient with my condition needs a lot of care. My home is fully adapted, but there wasn't enough care in the community for me to stay there. So I had to go to St Michael's. I miss home because I had a lovely garden. But my husband and children couldn't cope. I had some care but there wasn't enough. The care ended at 3pm, so I had no-one to help me if I got into difficulty after that.

I was diagnosed with MND six years ago. Before that, I had my own business as an holistic practitioner. My profession meant I was very in touch with my body and I knew something wasn't right.

When I was at work, I couldn't hold my pen. I would pick it up but I would just drop it. I knew it was wrong.

Initially, my doctor thought I might have been struggling because of the number of massages I gave people.

Then I went to a different doctor and she tested my reflexes and she knew something wasn't right. I had to wait 10 weeks for an appointment or pay £150 to go private so I paid the money.

When I went for the test, I knew the moment that I walked in that I had MND. But the doctor had to make sure. After all the tests, they gave me my formal diagnosis.

A lot of people don't know what MND is. My mum cried when I got my diagnosis. But I told her it would be alright. I had to be strong for my children, too.

I have always been busy, particularly looking after my children. I have a big family, many of my children are in the armed forces, and I love them a lot. They keep me going. The normal life span for MND is just over a year, but I've been going for more than six years.

'After I'd got my diagnosis, I changed the way I lived. wanted to make the most of life.'

After I'd got my diagnosis, I decided to change the way I lived. I ate what I wanted and decided to go where I wanted. I went travelling and crammed a lot in while I still could. I wanted to make the most of life. I went to Norway and Finland and Iceland, which were beautiful. I also went all around the Mediterranean and I loved Italy and France. I enjoyed travelling, I'm glad that I did.

I still picture all of those places in my memory.

Every birthday, I make sure I have a party, too. Life is for living.

My illness puts a strain on things. My husband

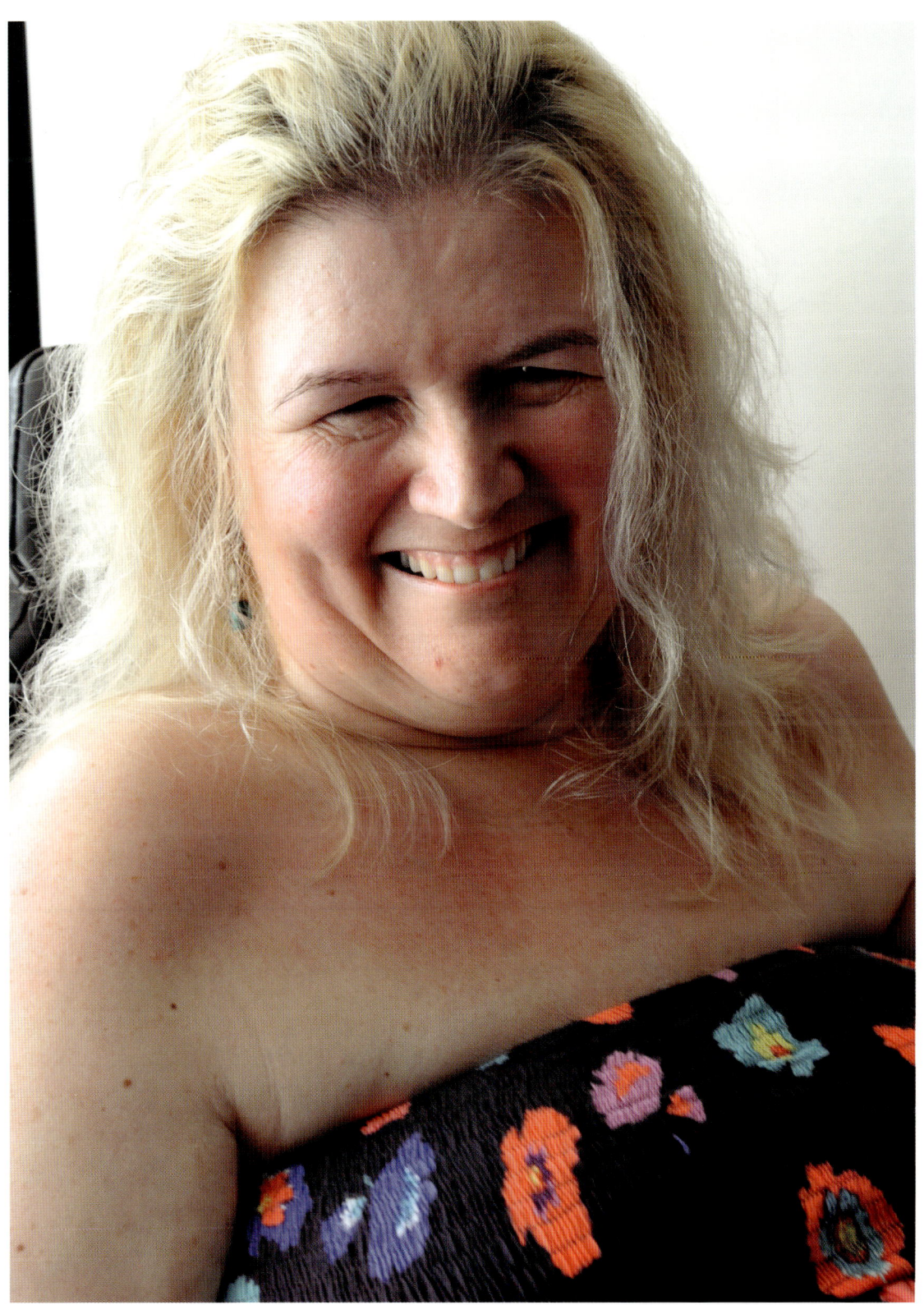

and I have found it difficult and sometimes things haven't been good. But that's his problem, not mine. I just try to live each day. I'm very determined to stay healthy and I only take one tablet a day.

MND is a frustrating illness because it slows everything down. I have to be very patient with people, too. I was a bit mad because the system meant I had to have a test to check my mental health. But I did the tests and the man had never met anyone who could do his tests so quickly.

The worst thing is that people see the wheelchair and they think you are incapable, they judge me. Everybody does. People ask the nurses the first question, rather than me. People don't even realise they are doing it. Everyone does it. But I tell them off. It's about a lack of education and a lack of knowledge. I don't blame the person, but I usually tell them to go and read up about it. I don't let it hurt me. I have more important things to be hurt by.

Even Gary Barlow, from Take That, did it. He came to the hospice and I told him off at St Michael's. He laughed. I asked: 'Gary, do you know what MND is?' I put him on the spot. He didn't know. So I told him: 'You're a naughty boy. I shall get your PA to look it up'.

He gave me a ticket to a Take That concert and it was incredible. I really enjoyed it. I've been to a lot of them and that was great; I was in the right place and had a great view.

I think that the mental side of things comes down to yourself and to the people you surround yourself with. I don't let negative people past the door. I only have positive people past the door.

St Michael's helps with that. The new building is wonderful, I prefer it to the old one because it's lovely.

As people, you can't fault them. They are very caring. I think people also forget it's a charity and that it needs support from the general public.

It all comes down to education. People need to know more about it.

Some people are very poorly when they go to the hospice. No one wants to die, but if they have hope and good care then the process is easier.

MND is a terrible disease because it affects the muscles. My body is killing itself. My brain is great, but my muscles are not. The muscles waste away and there is no cure. They don't know why it happens. It normally affects healthy people and fit people. A lot more men suffer than women. All of the essential organs are made from muscle, but they deteriorate and that means you eventually die. Your tongue is a muscle, too, and that deteriorates, so it becomes very difficult to talk. But MND can affect people differently. There are no rules. It's one-by-one, case-by-case.

On bad days, I have to block it out. I can't change it so I think of other things. I think of Norway or my children.

But you have to keep on fighting. If you give up, it will beat you, so you can't give up.

One of the biggest problem is fatigue and tiredness. The loss of dignity is also a problem. I'm afraid that has long gone.

I still look forward, even though I'm poorly. A lot of people say they have a bucket list. I don't really have one. For me, it's more about making sure that if I can do something I do it. I am limited, so I live within my capabilities.

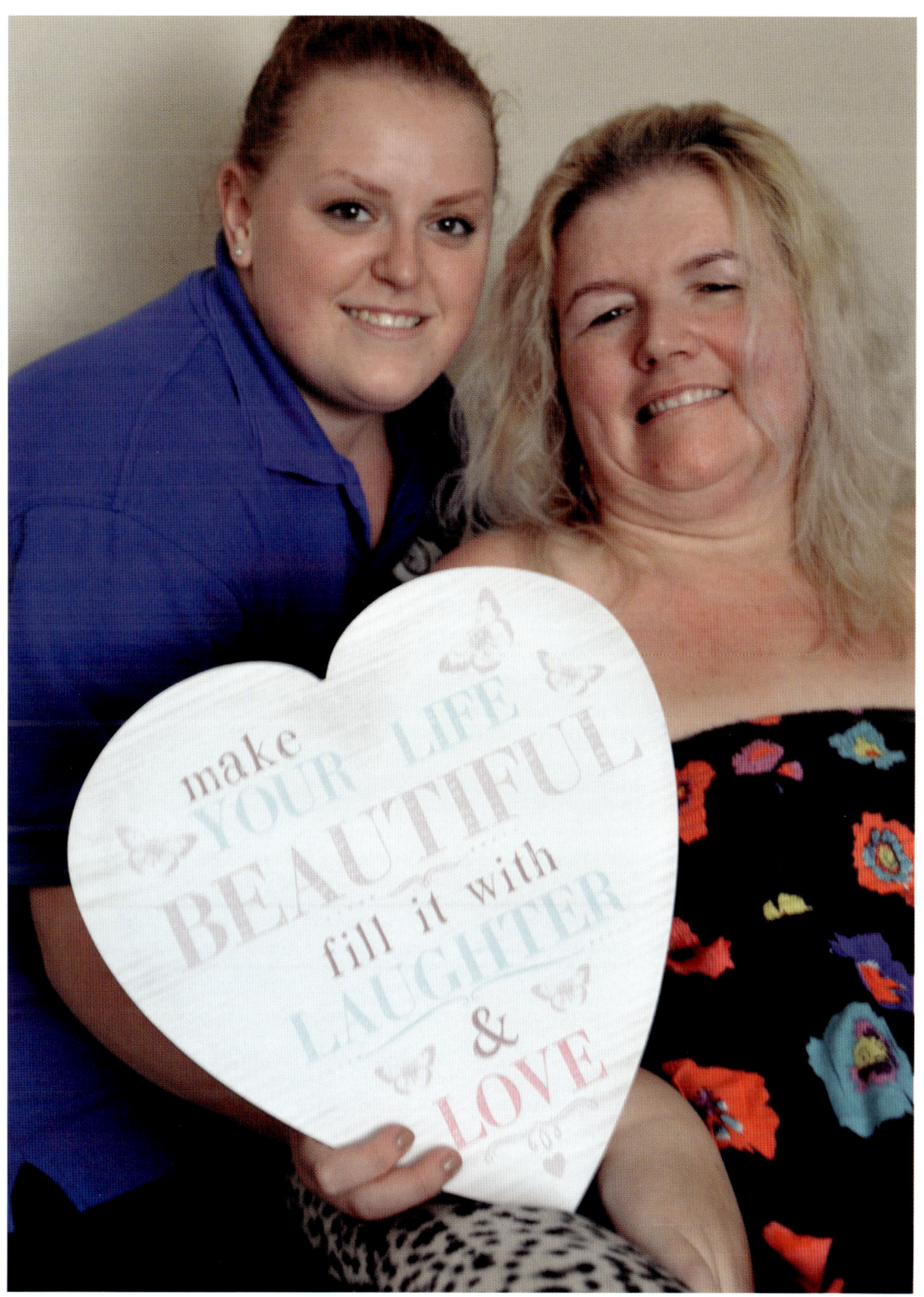

Mike Sloan, 57, Eardisley

My name's Mike, Mike Sloan, that's Sloan without an 'e'. I've been coming to the hospice for a while now. I'm still a young man, well, a middle-aged man; I'm not yet 60. I retired earlier this year through ill health.

I'd worked for most of my life as an engineer for BT. I spent 35 years with them, the last 20 as an electrical engineer. I moved to Hereford 20 years ago, in 1995, though the main reason was that I'd been divorced and wanted to get out the way and move on. I found myself a job at Madley and I was there for 20 years.

We used to climb telecoms masts that were over 800ft, it was all part of the job. We'd go up to Rugby Radio Station, which was on the top of a hill. There was an 850ft high mast and it was on the top of a hill, so it seemed even further. It was a bit nerve-wracking to start off with. But once I'd get beyond 50-60ft, I'd lose my reference, and then it would just be a climb. The view would get better and better, the higher I went. Of course, I'd have to make sure I didn't drop anything. If I dropped a tool from that height I'd never find it. We'd always park the van away from the mast, just in case; we didn't want to drop a tool and watch it embed itself in the roof. I really enjoyed my work, to be honest with you. It was the sort of job where you had to enjoy it because if you didn't you'd have problems. The work was very specialised.

Not all the masts were 850ft, some were quite a bit lower. And then some of the circular antennae were only 120ft high. But to get on top of those was different, they were actually far more dangerous. You are hooked on in three

separate places, but if you slipped and knocked yourself out you'd be in trouble. The fire brigade had a policy not to rescue you, we had our own emergency rescue teams, which we were all part of. It was good work and it kept me fit; I was 16-stone of muscle.

Away from work, my passions were cars and doing up houses; I did up four homes in 20 years. Unfortunately, I've not been able to do as much work to the present one as I'd have liked because of my condition, but my wife's brother, Giovanni, has come along and decorated for me. He did the place from top to bottom in four days, and did the carpets. That's family for you. He said he'd do it as a late wedding present because we got married last year. He did the whole house. I've got a new 20x25 garage for me, it'll be a place to stick all my cars; I've got four Minis.

I mentioned getting married last year and that was to Elisa, who is adorable. How did we meet? Well, it's amazing what you can pick up in Sainsbury's! I shouldn't laugh because it's an absolutely true story. Elisa, funnily enough, works for a cancer charity, for Marie Curie. She was doing an awareness day in the foyer in Sainsbury's, at Hereford, with a colleague of hers. I never normally use the store because I lived out at Drovers Barn, in Whitney-on-Wye. But it was a one-off. I needed fuel and a few bits and bobs so I went because I knew I'd be able to get everything in one place.

I walked in and there was a young lady stood in the foyer with the biggest beaming smile I'd ever seen in my life. I thought 'she looks alright'. We sort of clapped eyes on each other and she smiled even more. She came over and asked for a quick talk and that was it. Both of us just went 'wow'. And we've not been separated since. That was November 29, 2010.

She signed me up to Marie Curie and then I went to do my shopping. It was the usual sort of shop, I went round in a daze and ended up with

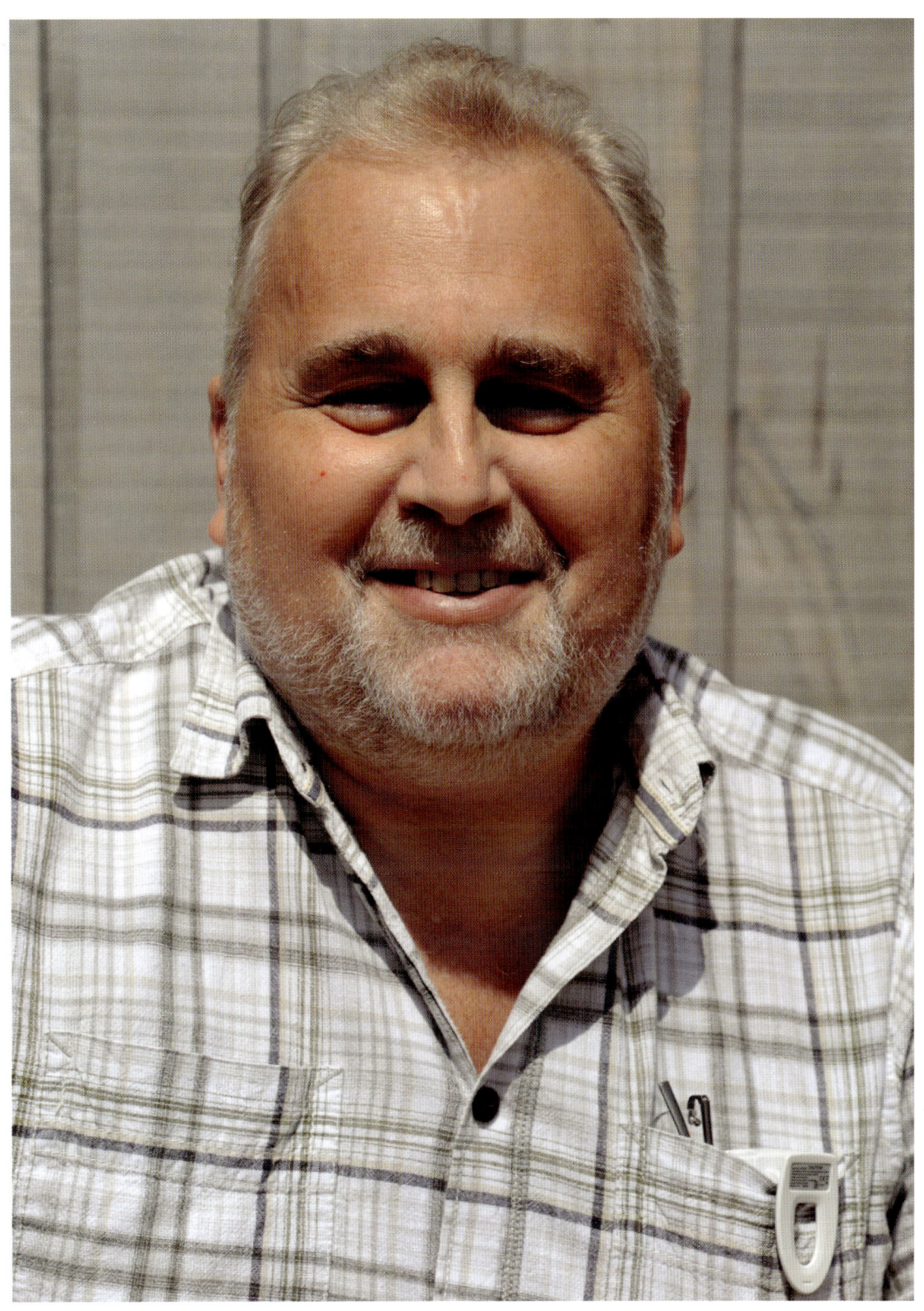

none of the things I'd gone in for. On my way out, we chatted again. I told Elisa: 'If you're ever up in Hereford again, give me a call and we'll go for a coffee'. I gave her my number and that was that. She kept me waiting a while. But then, two weeks later, I was in the kitchen at home one day and the phone went. It was Elisa. She said it was a personal call, nothing to do with work. We arranged to go for a meal on New Year's Eve and that was our proper first date. She drove all the way from Cwmbran, it was quite a trek, and when I arrived, she had her phone out and was trying to ring me. She was wearing a red coat and her face went scarlet when she saw me. She was more than a little flustered.

We got married last year, in 2014. I'd proposed about six months earlier, around the time of her birthday. I'd had my diagnosis so we got the family together for the weekend, with Elisa's sister and all the kids and a few friends. They came on the Sunday and her birthday was the Tuesday. I got everybody together, quietly, in the lounge. I said to her: 'I suppose I'd better make you Mrs Sloan'. It took her totally by surprise. She was sort of expecting a proposal a few days later on her birthday. So she sat there with her mouth wide open, but she did say yes, so it wasn't all bad. That was in the August and we got married in the May.

The wedding was superb, absolutely brilliant. We lived in Breinton, down by the river, in an old vicarage. We wanted to get married in the church, but we weren't sure if the vicar would let us. We went to see him and said: 'Look, we're not first-time-rounders. We're both second-or-third-

time-rounders.' We asked: 'What's the chance of getting married in the church?'

The vicar told us there were a couple of rules. He asked if we'd had anything to do with each other's divorces and asked whether we lived together and so on. We got through those questions and he said there was no problem.

We needed to set a date and Elisa thought it would be a nice idea to get married on the anniversary of my father's death, which was May 4, 2005. My dad, George, had always had a saying: 'May the fourth be with you'. She thought it would be nice to honour his memory, you know, to turn a negative into a positive and make a nice memory.

On our wedding day, I basically walked to church. It was down the road from the house. Lisa wanted an old-fashioned car so my best man, Scotty, managed to get us a 1929 Rolls Royce from a guy he knew. Before the service, Elisa went for a drive with Scotty's brother-in-law. There was no point in just driving from the house to the church because it was only down the road, so Elisa drove round the village and ended up being 20 minutes late. It was a wonderful day and everybody was thrilled to bits.

> 'Elisa thought it would be a nice idea to get married on the anniversary of my father's death'

The weather was like it is today; absolutely beautiful. There wasn't a cloud in the sky. The vicar inserted a lot of humour and made sure we knew what we were committing ourselves to. After the ceremony, we took a ride from the church to the Railway Inn, at Dinmore, via Sainsbury's car park, where we'd met. It was a Sunday, so there weren't millions of people there, fortunately.

We'd had a holiday before, a pre-honeymoon. And we went to Lanzarote too, afterwards. We were planning a trip to the British Grand Prix, too, but that fell through because I wasn't well enough. And from then onwards, it's been a fantastic life with Elisa.

Elisa was the one who knew I was unwell. I'd felt poorly for a while, back in June 2013, and she encouraged me to see the doctor. I had all sorts of scans over a two-week period to find out what was wrong. Then one day, during that two-week period, Elisa took me to hospital. She thought I looked like a dying man. She'd worked in residential care, a long time ago, so she'd sat with people who were dying. It was just a look that she recognised. She didn't like it. So she said: 'How do you feel about me taking you to A&E for a check?' I said okay.

It was all diagnosed from there, really. They measured me on the Gleason score and I got nine/10, which is the late stages of cancer. 10 is the maximum.

Now I know I ought to tell you I was shocked and devastated, but I wasn't. It sounds strange to say it, but I was totally relieved when I got my diagnosis. I'd been tested for gallstones and kidney stones and IBS and they'd ruled everything out. So I was thinking: 'If I haven't got those, what have I got?' In the back of my mind, I'd worried about whether I'd got cancer.

When we were in A&E, there were a lot of people running about. They asked how much I drank because my liver score was through the roof; they thought I was an alcoholic. The final test was the PSA test, which measures the protein given out by the prostate. A normal score is between 0-10. Anything above 10 is possibly cancerous. Mine was 1,270.

My first question was simple and immediate. I asked: 'Can you do anything about it?' They said they could treat it but added that my score was so high that there was probably little chance of curing it. So I asked them whether it would kill me. They told me prostate cancer wouldn't kill me, but secondary cancers might. They said when the cancer spreads, that's when you've got problems. And my score was so high that the cancer had almost certainly spread.

As I said, I was okay with it. I'd felt so poorly that it was a relief to know what I'd got and that they could do something about it. I realised I might not survive it, but at least I had hope and at least I had a little extra time to sort myself out and live. You know, I'd got the opportunity to get my head right and come to terms with things. When you have cancer, the mental battle is one of the biggest, probably even more so than physical.

Now don't get me wrong. I'm not saying it's easy to deal with, physically. Believe me, it's not. When I get up in the morning, I have pain in my leg. But I know I have to move, I have to get up for my ablutions. And that's when it tends to kick off. Getting out of the bed in the morning is the hardest part of the day. Each day, the pain changes. I got up this morning and the background pain was two out of 10 and the stabbing pain was six to seven out of 10. On some

'I'd felt so poorly that it was a relief to know what I'd got and that they could do something about it.'

days, it can literally go beyond the 10 scale. I've had the odd day where I've gone to move and the pain has been so acute that I've not been able to. It's felt like somebody sticking daggers in me, it's been that bad. It's genuinely been beyond the point of tolerable, it really has. I've literally been sat here crying with pain. The staff at St Michael's have to give me an injection of morphine, straight into my arm. They give me a muscle relaxant as well. Then you just have to sit there and wait for it to wear off, there's nothing you can do. When the pain strikes, that's it. Elisa will sit here, holding my hand, offering verbal support. She'll do whatever she can. At the moment, Elisa has a bed here with me, at the hospice, and she stays 24-7, unless I have a visitor.

I stay positive. I stay focused. The hospice helps with that. This place is all about giving people the best quality of life possible. They keep me out of pain and help me to stay positive. But I think I contribute to that because I've always been a positive person. There's no point moping. If I did that, the cancer would grab me and have me and I don't want that, that's the last thing on my mind.

Like I said, the mental battle is the hardest one to win. You never forget you have the disease. It's always there at the back of your mind. But I tend to not give it room in my mind, I just push it out. You know that it will come along to remind you it's there; it'll stab you in the leg. And I think: 'Yeah, thanks a lot'. But once you've got over that discomfort with meditation or medication, you move on.

I filter out the anger and frustration. I know I've got a terminal illness, but I still have so much to live for and so many people that I want to be with. What's the point thinking about the disease? I'd rather get on with it, I'd rather try to be happy and make the best of things. I can potter around with my cars, be with Elisa or spend time with my family instead. I've got a bucket list, too. There are silly things, you know, like going down to WH Smith and buying a magazine because there's an article I want to read. Then there are bigger things: next week, we're going to see the guitarist Joe Bonamassa in concert in Cardiff. It'll be a long day and a hard day but I'm determined to do it. I'll take whatever medication is required and I'll need medication on the way back, but I won't quit. My bucket list has lots of things that I need to do as well as things that I just want to do. There's a list in between, of the things I'd like to do. It depends how things pan out. You just have to do the things you can when you feel well enough. And if they're not possible on any given day, then, you know, you say: 'That's alright, there's always tomorrow'.

One of the things that gives me the most pleasure is my collection of Mini cars. I've got four. The latest edition has been nicknamed The Green Hornet. I showed Elisa a photograph of it before I bought it and she just told me to go and buy it. So I went down to Brighton, with Elisa's son, Nathan, and picked it up. It's a real beast, proper old school. It's got a 2-litre 16-valve engine in it with 178bhp. It goes like the proverbial rocket. It scares everybody that goes out in it. The first time I took Elisa out, she got out after and said: 'If you think I'm going out again in that, you've got another think coming'.

> ## 'There's no point moping. If I did that, the cancer would grab me and have me and I don't want that'

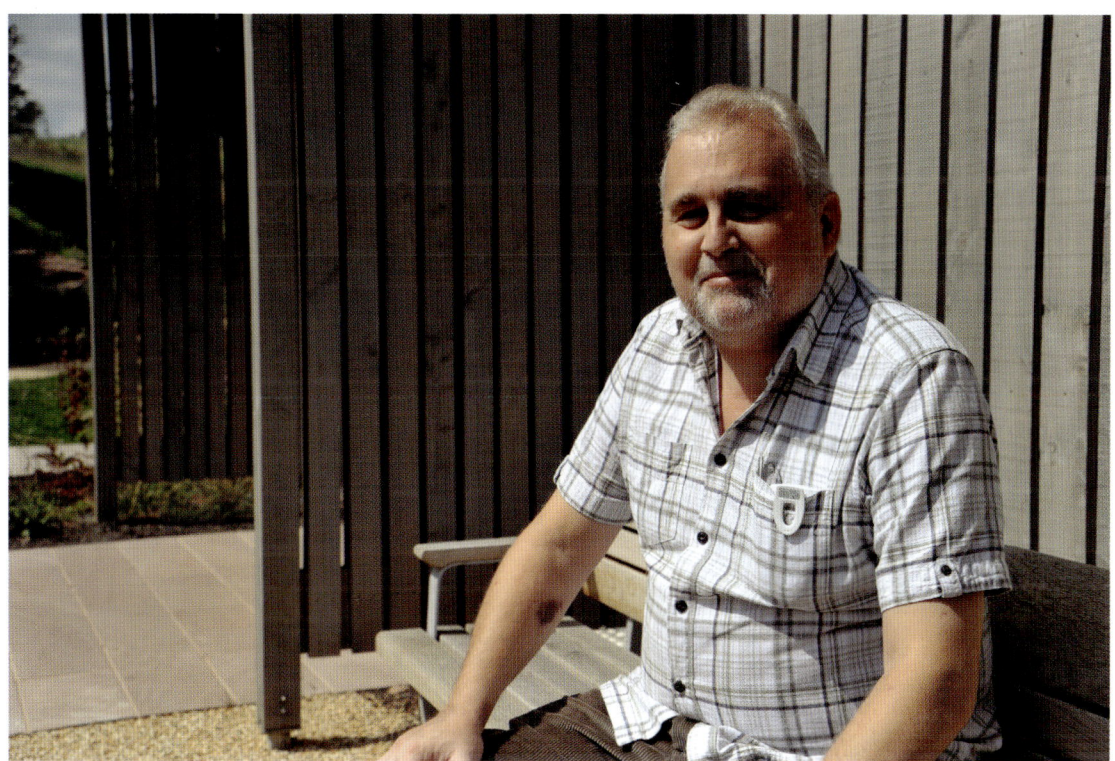

Her sons were all watching and they were rolling about on the floor, laughing their heads off.

Elisa and I do what we can. We went to see The Who not so long ago, in Cardiff. They were good, except they all had colds and two-thirds of the way through Roger Daltry lost his voice. It didn't matter though because we were in Wales. The male voice choir helped him out and everybody sang the words for them. Music is a real passion. I used to be in bands for 10 years, I was a rocker with long hair and 27-inch flares.

I use different methods to ease the pain. Reiki is one of the most effective. I have two younger brothers and the youngest is named Paul, he's 10 years younger than me. He and his wife are both reiki masters and teachers as well. They've been to see me quite a few times and when they come down they usually perform reiki on me. I have it here at the hospice, too, and at a day centre in Hereford. But when I receive it from Paul or his wife, it's far more potent. I don't know whether that's psychological or not but they certainly make things a lot easier for me. The feelings of relief and elation are profound. Reiki calms everything down, it clears my mind.

There are times, though, when even that doesn't work. And a few weeks ago I went through my roughest patch so far. I had what I can only describe as an out-of-body experience. I was at home and both my brothers were down. It might sound strange, but on one of those particular days, my mind had a day out from my body. I'll explain. I was sitting in the lounge with my middle brother, Phil, and just before lunch, I sort of went out on a little trip on my own, so to speak. Basically, my consciousness sort of left my body. It was as if my body was sat in the chair and I was in a white room. I was in two places at the same time. I was aware of my body but my mind was somewhere else.

I can remember it vividly. I was in a pure white room and I could see myself lying on the settee, even though I was actually sitting there. My consciousness was halfway up an invisible staircase in this pure white room. Everything was so white you couldn't make out the edges. I was looking up towards the sky, to my left-hand side, and that was white as well.

My body was in a lot of pain at the time, a hell of a lot of pain, and I didn't really know whether I wanted to be with my body or separate from it. I was curious as to why I was in the room. I didn't understand the reason for it. I sensed that if I looked upwards I might see people from my past, people who'd already died. I've seen my late parents before, for instance, after they'd died. They came to see me at home. It was like a vision, or whatever you want to call it.

So on that particular day, I was in this white room and I was sort of thinking: 'Am I halfway between life and death. Am I really in that space?' I was looking at my body on the sofa thinking: 'That is in so much pain that I don't really want to be there'. And then I was aware that I was still in the white room and I was thinking: 'Do I want to go back, or do I want to carry on?' Curiosity got the better of me. I thought: 'If I do go up those stairs, will I get back?' I was waiting for somebody to open a door at the top, anybody, my father, stepmum, grandparents, a child I lost when we were young. If somebody had just opened the door and said: 'Come on, you'll be safe, come with us', I'd have possibly gone. I can't say definitely. I wasn't afraid, I was just curious. I thought to myself: 'If I go forward and decide to make that commitment, is the living part over? Is life over? Will my body just die away'. And I waited and waited and waited and nobody came. I got to the point where I thought: 'If I take another step and nothing happens, is there a dividing line that I can't see? Will I still be able to return to the living world?' I wasn't ready to die, I didn't want to

leave the physical world, but I didn't want to be in that amount of pain either. So I wondered which would be the best for everybody, to be honest. If I carried on, I knew I would be out of pain and I'd hopefully be with my family. But I couldn't guarantee that because nobody came. So after hours of thinking, it became a case of: 'Right, I haven't got the answer I was after, so I'll step back into the living world'.

In the meantime, Elisa had been trying to wake me up. She thought I was just sleeping. The whole thing went on for hours and hours and while it was happening I was trying to analyse it and make sense of what I should do. I knew that if I went back, I'd be in a state of catatonic pain. So for a while, I wondered if it was best to just slip away quietly. But I wasn't ready, I didn't really want to. It wasn't the right time.

That experience changed my outlook on life. I became more determined than ever to stay alive. I became even more positive. Despite what life throws at me, however much pain I'm in, I've just got to get on with it and do it.

My relationships changed, too. I realised that some of the people who I had expected to be there for me seemed to have every excuse under the sun not to be there. But the people who I didn't think I could necessarily count on were all there, they really came to the fore. For me, of course, the main person was Elisa. She's never wavered. She's been upset and down, obviously, but that's normal. We comfort each other.

The disease impacts on everything. Take my mum, Hazel, for instance; she's struggling because she's 78, she's got me ill and my brother is ill too. She's not just my mum, she's my best mate as well. She's the sort of woman you can talk to. She's got this attitude: 'Just get on with it'. She's always been like that and it's rubbed off on me.

I think a lot about her and I also think about my grandfather, George. He was a right old devil. He was from Wrexham, in north Wales, and he had a Presbyterian background. He managed to get himself mixed up with a married woman and he moved to Yorkshire, the year my dad was born. My dad was the result of the slight indiscretion, shall we say. George had been a miner in Wales and got a job as a miner in Doncaster. He lost a leg in a pit accident but he soldiered on. He used to say: 'Listen lad, if you worry, you die. If you don't worry, you die. It's the same either way, so what are you worried for?'

And he was right. These days, I don't see any point in worrying. If something is out of your control, and my disease is, all I can do is take the medication and get on with it. If that's the option that you've got, you've got to go with it. It's difficult because everything they give you has an effect. You have to manage the side effects. But you get on with it. That philosophy from my grandfather, and particularly from my mum, carries me through. That's the way I was brought up. If I've got a problem, I've just got to deal with it. There's no point in sitting round moping, thinking about the things I can or can't do.

Look, I know I'm ill, but that doesn't mean I don't think about the future. The fact that I have a terminal illness changes nothing. I still have to have a goal in life. There's lots I still want to do. I accept some things are impossible, but I look at the things I might be able to do. I'm not going to race fast cars round circuits any more because my body won't take it, I'd still love to do it and the thought is still there, but I know I can't do it. Perhaps one day, there'll be a miracle and let's be positive: I hope there is. But if there isn't, that's

'. . . for a while, I wondered if it was best to just slip away quietly. But I wasn't ready.'

tough. You have to accept it for what it is. I've done a lot of things in my younger days. I've lived a good life and I'm still trying to live a good life.

The people at St Michael's make my life so much better than it would otherwise be. Being here is like being in a four star hotel, it's absolutely brilliant. It doesn't matter what you want, they do their best to help you. You come in here for a reason and they're never intrusive. They care, they really do, they just come along and chat to you.

I see a psychologist on a Thursday, a guy called Ray, and he's the type who is a typical psychologist: he never tells you a thing but he gives you a million things to think about. He'll see how I am then he'll go down a particular line and give me something to think about. He helps me to formulate a response to what's going on. He's not the only one. The nurses are just as incredible. They're open and honest. This morning, the nurse came in and asked what our plans were. I told them I wanted to go home but I'd got pain in my leg. So the nurse said that was no problem. She said: 'If you set your mind to going home, just keeping thinking about that and we'll deal with any pain or any other issues you have'. They told me to keep being positive about going home. They say: 'Focus on thinking that you're going home. Don't think you can't do it'. And so that's the way I think. My body tunes into that positive line of thought. And, funnily enough, the pain has stopped completely.

Ann Jellyman, 60
Eardisley

I was born in South Africa and I moved to England 15 years ago. During that time, I've worked all over the UK. My job was in domiciliary care. When I was growing up, I didn't imagine my journey would bring me here.

I was born in Bloemfontein, in South Africa. My father had moved there after the Second World War. We stayed there until I was nine or 10 and then we moved to Port Elizabeth. After school, I went to do a teaching degree, but at the end of that I didn't want to teach. I joined the hotel industry against my parents' wishes. I did my in-service training and spent almost 20 years in the hotel industry. That was during a remarkable time in global politics because South Africa was an apartheid state.

Working in hotels in those years was extremely difficult because of the terrorist threat from the ANC. There were constant bomb alerts and dealings with the security police. At the hotels in which I worked we looked after high-level political visitors, from presidents through to diplomats. It was an unbelievable career, it really and truly was.

My role was to be a liaison for the security police. If there were any bomb threats or warning calls, I would have to keep the person on the phone long enough for the police to trace the call. If there was any baggage left unattended, I was the one who would have to call the right people in to dispose of it. It was really hectic. The hotels that I worked at were the ones that had the highest dignitaries.

After the Apartheid era quietened down, the unions started. There were a lot of strikes and riots and everything. It didn't ever seem to stop. There were days when we would operate a hotel with no staff because the workers were so intimidated that they wouldn't come to work. Guests still arrived to stay at the hotel and we used to have to be very versatile, working the kitchens and housekeeping and everything else: the show had to go on. I loved my career. I was known as the drama queen because if anything was ever going to happen it was when I was on duty.

We had many evacuations. I was always the last person to evacuate because I would be talking on the phone and having to wait for clearance from the security police. It was real MI5 stuff. They would want to have a confirmed link to the bombers and where they were talking from. We had the Israeli President stay with us for a while. On another occasion, the Iranian embassy was closed for a while so their staff stayed in the hotel. It was a real high profile, topical thing. You think 'my goodness, I lived through that'.

Before Nelson Mandela was released from prison, I was headhunted by the education department in South Africa to work in a university. They wanted me to help oversee the language change from Afrikaans to English. There were a lot of riots because students were fighting against colonial involvement, which I could understand. But then they had to understand that if the colonials had not got there, the country would not have had what it had become. The British left a valuable heritage behind and taught people a lot of valuable things. It was a case of co-existence, really.

The students were very violent. They would come into the administration office and stand on the desks and kick and trash the computers while we were working. It was far worse than anything I ever experienced in the hotel industry, and that was when I was dealing with terrorists.

Around 1989/90, I decided I'd had enough of all the stress and pressure. We'd changed the

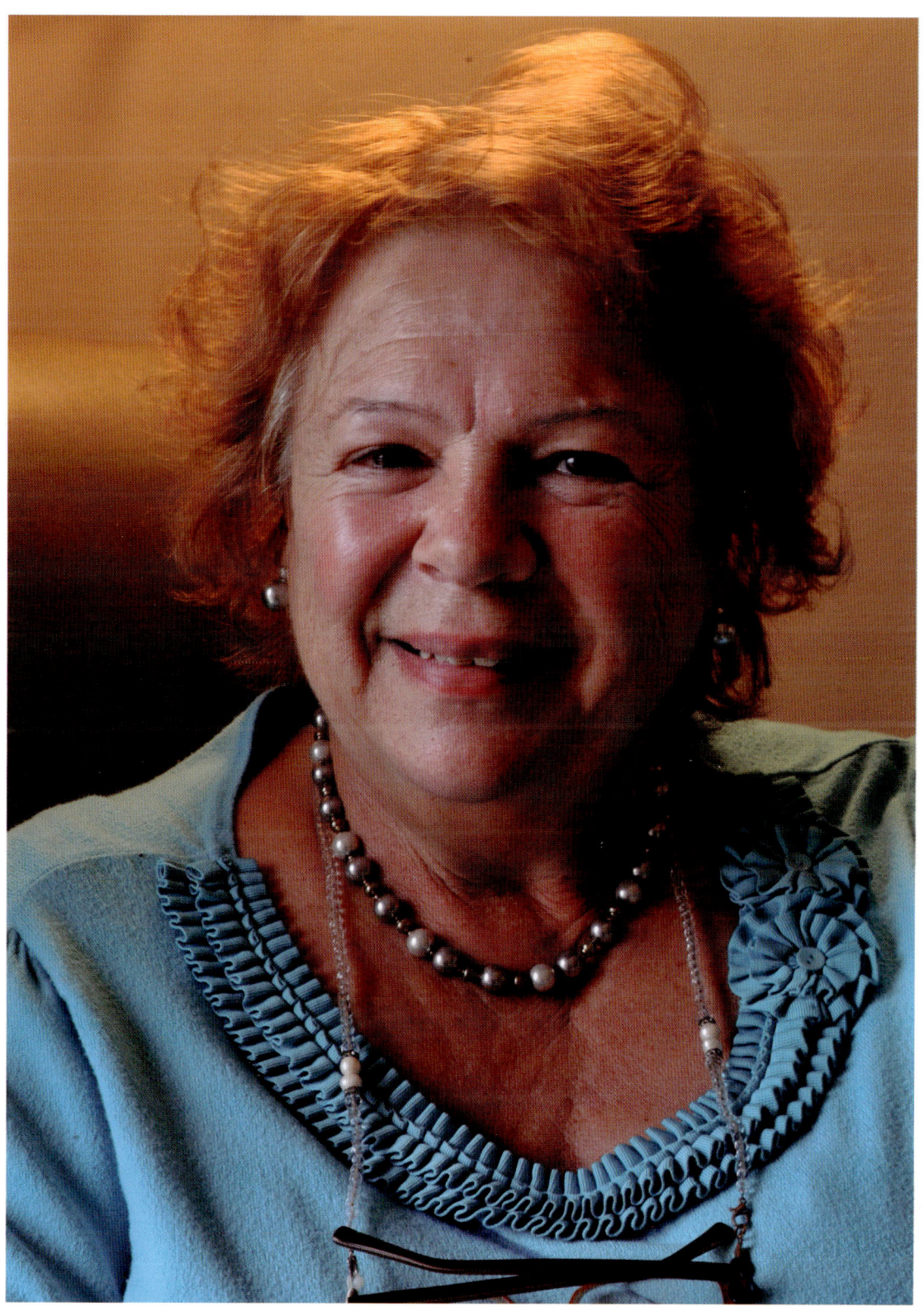

education programme and I remember a couple of students who were being intimidated by their fellow black students, which I couldn't quite understand. I remember two in particular, who were suffering unjust treatment. One little girl's father had been murdered in the mines and she had no other living relatives. Then there was a young black man from Ghana who was a brilliant student. He studied electrical engineering and ended up of his own accord studying Japanese and going on to work for Toyota. I took both of them under my wing and was proud of them for pulling themselves up and doing something better with their lives. They gave me a lot of hope for the African continent.

Around that time, I decided I wanted to move out of South Africa and I looked at Canada and Australia and the USA but nothing felt quite right, so I went back to South Africa and decided to open my own business. Before I could, I was headhunted again by Continental Tyres and I started travelling. I led a very international lifetime. It was my time to spread my wings. My father passed away around that time and I was on the road for a number of years, doing a lot of TV work for Continental and managing the advertising and public relations. I would be away for weeks on end. It was quite hectic, but a very nice job that I really enjoyed.

My father had led an interesting life himself. He was a photojournalist. His name was John Jellyman and he did a lot of work for the newspapers, capturing life in South Africa. It was remarkable.

He did a lot of photographs and worked for mission stations. We had many Christmases on the missions. When we moved to Port Elizabeth, he worked for Donald Woods, the anti-apartheid activist who was the editor of the Daily Dispatch and was known for befriending fellow activist Steve Biko. From a security point of view, things got a little tight. My father did a lot of photojournalism work with Donald and it was a huge learning curve. We were able to see different aspects of the situation that had developed in South Africa at that time. I had a good grounding of what was right and wrong.

In my own career, I reached a glass ceiling with Continental Tyres that I couldn't push through, so I opened my own public relations company and did a lot of work for General Motors and other big clients. Then the opportunity came for me to move over here, to the UK. The South African government was starting a black empowerment scheme and I was expected to take on two black people and give them director status, with director salaries, even though they didn't have to bring in any work. I couldn't justify that, so I sold my business and decided to pack up and move over here.

I'd worked in business all of my life and wanted to do something completely different and contribute to society, that's why I went into the care industry. I felt I had a lot to give to the elderly who couldn't get out. I worked for two agencies and cared for people in their own homes.

Things were all fine until 2014. By then, I was looking forward to my 60th birthday but I became ill. I had problems with my gall bladder and the

'As a carer, I'd always been looking out for other people but nobody was looking out for me.'

doctors decided it should be removed. That was in June 2014. They opted to remove the gall bladder because they were concerned I would develop gall stones. I was put on medication afterwards, though it had very bad side effects. I'll tell you more about those in a moment.

After the operation, I had constant check-ups but I was diagnosed on the 8th of January 2015 with gall bladder cancer. Unfortunately for me I wasn't aware of anything being wrong, so when the diagnosis came through it really hit me badly from a psychological point of view. Having worked away from home most of the time I never really built up a connection with people in and around where I lived. So for me it was extremely difficult trying to find a bit of normal humanity and being in a caring environment. I had no family and only a few close friends. From a psychological point of view I just had a complete traumatic breakdown. I was given two weeks to get my affairs in order. It was a huge shock. I was at that time still working so I had to give up my job. I had to explain why I was stopping work and try and get a whole lot of things organised. I went from feeling fine and looking forward to turning 60 to absolutely having my life turned upside down and not knowing how long I had got. I didn't know if I had got enough time to sort things out or not. It was very traumatic.

The problems with my medication made things worse. I basically went until October 2015 suffering a continual allergic reaction before I took the decision myself to stop taking my medicine. The minute I stopped the medication, all my symptoms disappeared. For me, that gave me a new lease of life. While I was feeling rotten and sick, I couldn't see the light. That's why coming here to the hospice helped me so much. I had so many people I could talk to at the hospice who were sympathetic and understanding and who helped me from a support point of view.

In retrospect, I now realise that the pain

and everything I was experiencing wasn't the reaction to the cancer, it was the reaction to the medication.

The drugs that I was on after weren't cancer-related, they were just an antacid. But they made me feel like I had eaten rotten eggs, I had a constant sulphur reflux. The pain was coming from under the liver area and I assumed it was the gall bladder. Only when I stopped the medication did those symptoms go. Now, I can eat anything I want. Up until then I couldn't.

As a carer, I'd always been looking out for other people but nobody was looking out for me. After being told to sort out my affairs I did the best I could. But there comes a point where you just hit a brick wall. It is difficult to get things done when you are feeling so sick and so vulnerable. If I didn't have people here at the hospice to help and point me in the right direction, I wouldn't know what to do.

The cancer diagnosis in January hit me hard. The surgeon told me that because of the nature of the cancer, the prognosis was not good. The lymph gland closest to the gall bladder had also been removed when I had my gall bladder taken out and they feared that the cancer might have spread further. My surgeon told me I had a rare cancer and there was no guaranteed remedy, not chemo or anything. I would have been in a hit and miss situation and there would have been no guarantee about my quality of life. So I opted not to have treatment. I thought if I was going to be alive for such a short space of time, why would I make things more miserable? I didn't want to do that, just from a self-preservation point of view. I'm now pleased that I didn't seek treatment. It's helped me with a lot of things, particularly my acceptance of what's happened.

As things stand, they don't know what my life expectancy is. Initially, they gave me two weeks to get my affairs in order. I pushed them in a corner and asked how long it would be for me to be physically capable and they told me two weeks. So I could have died within a fortnight. That was back in January 2015. It was devastating. I couldn't sleep. I just cried all the time. I didn't want to tell anybody about my diagnosis. I didn't want people feeling sorry for me. The trouble with me telling others is that some people don't know how to deal with you so they back off. That's exactly what has happened and that was my fear. You know your friends pretty well and you know who can take what. The two that I didn't want to tell have actually backed off. They've told me to keep in touch and I can send an email but I get nothing back. People are scared, they don't know how to speak about it and don't know what to say. I've lost those two particular people now as friends. The relationships have changed irreparably, which is genuinely tragic.

That was the reason for my reluctance in talking about it. The two people who are my next of kin got such a shock. They ask you all the questions that you can't answer. You haven't had the chance to answer them yet because you are so traumatised. So you can't give anybody the right information anyway. It was a very, very traumatic time for me before I started coming to the hospice.

At Macmillan, the oncologist suggested that I see a particular doctor and he advocated that I try and find somewhere to go. I was for a while just holed up alone at home. I could not eat because of the reaction to the medication. I was flat on my back because of the medication. It was off the scale in terms of depression and anxiety. There was no point in opening my eyes in the morning.

The days were a question of the sun coming up and the sun going down. It was just a question of getting through the day. Much of the time, I just slept. I felt physically sick from the reaction to the medication, which wasn't working for me. I also became very dizzy. It wasn't picked up for over a year. I was almost rotten, basically. That's why I chose to come off the medication.

Since October, I have had no problems whatsoever. It's been a long haul but I've managed to get myself back up and on my feet again. As regards the hospice here, they've helped me a lot. Every time I had an attack or felt poorly, the nurses here would help me. They have pacified me and reassured me that things are not as bad as I might think they are.

The symptoms I experienced as a side effect from the drugs were the same as the ones I would have expected from the cancer. So, for instance, there was lethargy, dizziness, nausea, the loss of appetite. Everything that they told me about I experienced, but I thought it was from the cancer rather than the bad reaction to the drugs. I assumed the cancer was out of control and my life had been very much shortened. It was extremely difficult and the medical profession did not know what was wrong with me. I couldn't work out what was going on because I felt so lousy. It was an awful situation and nobody knew what to do, including the medical profession. But the staff at the hospice were my back-up. Coming on a Friday for a reflexology treatment or a massage was so invaluable, if only as a release of the tension. The only night of the week I would sleep well would be on a Friday night. It was like a breath of fresh air and it gave me space.

And then the hospice chaplain has been absolutely marvellous. The chapel here is a wonderful facility to have. I can talk and pray and have communion. That's a very nice aspect for me because most of the churches are shut today. You can't get to see somebody unless you book an appointment. It's very nice to have that facility on the premises instead of having to phone the parish to book an appointment to see the vicar. Sometimes, you don't want your congregation to know what's going on. I haven't told my own congregation because I don't want the reaction from them that I've had from my friends. You see, I'm the same person. But we are such social creatures that it's difficult. I'm not a psychologist or psychiatrist, but people do put labels on you, whether they mean to or not. I'm considered the 'friend with cancer'. It's very hush-hush among my friends. People talk. They need help as well, in coming to terms with what's happening with me. So you just realise that cancer has such negative connotations to it. The cancer word is terrible. People just don't know how to behave around you when you have cancer.

I don't think it's tiring any more. I've learned to push it to the side and pretend they're not talking about me. If you don't do that you're almost unable to participate in the conversation. People want to be sympathetic and ask after you. The people who ask in that way, however, aren't the people who are going to be there for the long haul. You instinctively know they'll fall away. That's the difference here at the hospice. They don't have to ask.

'The chapel here is a wonderful facility to have.'

They already know how you are. They can see from the way you look, the way you behave or the things you say. They treat you with a lot of respect and give you a lot of dignity.

You can be yourself at the hospice, you don't have to put up a brave face and be all happiness and bells and whistles. You can be yourself. It's immaterial. The hospice doesn't judge me. They don't try to put me in a box, you know: the okay box, or the poorly box or the upset box. They don't do that here. They are concerned, they do not leave any stone unturned.

In the beginning I was exceptionally emotional, as you can quite understand. They had a couple of workshops here and one of them was on death and dying. I don't think I heard one word of the entire workshop, I just cried all the way through.

I didn't have the physical energy to get up and remove myself from the room. What was so nice for me was that nobody looked at me. They just let me be. I was able to work my way through it, as sad as it was for me. They didn't look at me or try to get me out of there, they just accepted that I was upset. I was really grateful about that. There was no embarrassment on their part. They were very supportive. Sometimes, my tears are like a tap, they just come and I've no control over it.

They have helped in terms of accepting death because I have elected not to die at home alone. They are fully aware of my wishes and the fact that I have no family. My next of kin are friends. I don't want to put myself on them and burden their families. For me, that is very helpful. I have the medical assistance here too; there is nothing else I could want for. There is nowhere I would rather be.

I find the whole building so aesthetically peaceful, it's quite incredible. There is a vibe here that you can't put your finger on. It's not just peaceful or happy; it's all encompassing. It's nurturing, it's soulful and peaceful, it's everything to me. The outlook, the gardens, the views, the way the property has been developed: all of it is incredible. So much thought has gone into it. It's absolutely incredible. From the time you walk in, you feel okay. You don't feel as though it's an overwhelming experience. It's not what I expected from a hospice. I expected hospital beds and wards and pain and suffering. But there isn't. You don't see any of that. It's rather marvellous. The hospice is a blessing in disguise.

Brian Jones 67, Hereford

Well, where should I start? I guess with events that happened 11 weeks ago. I dislocated my shoulder. I got up in the night and I went across the room to put the light on. But I tripped and fell and that was it. Ouch. Flipping 'eck, it's been really painful ever since; it feels as though it's not getting better.

I got to the hospital and they put my shoulder back in but I can't bloomin' move it. I was praying to God when I was on the floor in the night that I hadn't broke my arm, but I almost wish I had broken it. It would have been easier. A dislocation can take a lot longer to heal than a break, apparently. It's taped up now, so that the muscles bind together. But it's been bad news for me because I'm right-handed.

I must be honest, it's been getting me down. There's my shoulder and my illness and I'm hopeless left-handed. I just have no control over what I'm doing. It makes me feel a bloody nuisance. I'll have been at the hospice for a month on Monday. I had to come in because I couldn't manage the stairs, I just couldn't cope in my house.

There's a lot that I haven't told you, so let me begin. I lost my wife 14 years ago, so I've been on my own a long time. My wife was in here, too. They looked after her well, they did. Thank God for these places.

As well as my shoulder, I have liver cancer and that's been dragging me down. Then I had an infection: c difficile, or something like that. I thought I'd just been feeling weak and run down but apparently I was really ill with c difficile. The doctor told me I was ill. They put me into an isolation unit in the hospice. I spent a fortnight just shut in. I hope to God the c difficile doesn't come back. I had it a couple of years ago, but I thought it was the side effects from the drugs.

Apparently the blessed thing hangs on in there, in the body, and it's a devil of a job to get rid of. But hopefully I've fought it off and we're on top of it.

I've been in bad shape for a while. I got my liver diagnosis two or three years ago. Time goes so quick, I can't remember exactly when. I'm not sure it's manageable, as such. I think it's been getting worse and I know I've only got so much time.

The way I found out about the cancer was a bit strange, to say the least. I'd had other problems before I got my diagnosis. I'd been under the doctor with a bowel problem and I had to have an operation to sort things out. When I came round after the bowel operation, the doctor told me not to worry. He said: 'The operation's gone super. The way you're going you'll live longer than me. It's gone 100%, it's super.' I kept going to see the surgeon after the operation for tests but there was something not quite right with my blood. My blood was elevated, or something. I didn't think too much of it and just carried on, as you do.

Then I was at the NEC one day: I was a coach driver and I had a coachload of people with me. My doctor rang me, not the surgeon, and over the phone he told me: he said: 'Brian, it could be cancer'. And I thought, 'Christ Almighty what are you telling me that for now?' I had a coachload of people with me at the NEC and how I drove the coach back I'll never know. I thought surely a specialist should have got me in and told me that. But there you are: my doctor called and told me over the phone.

It really knocked me the way they went about

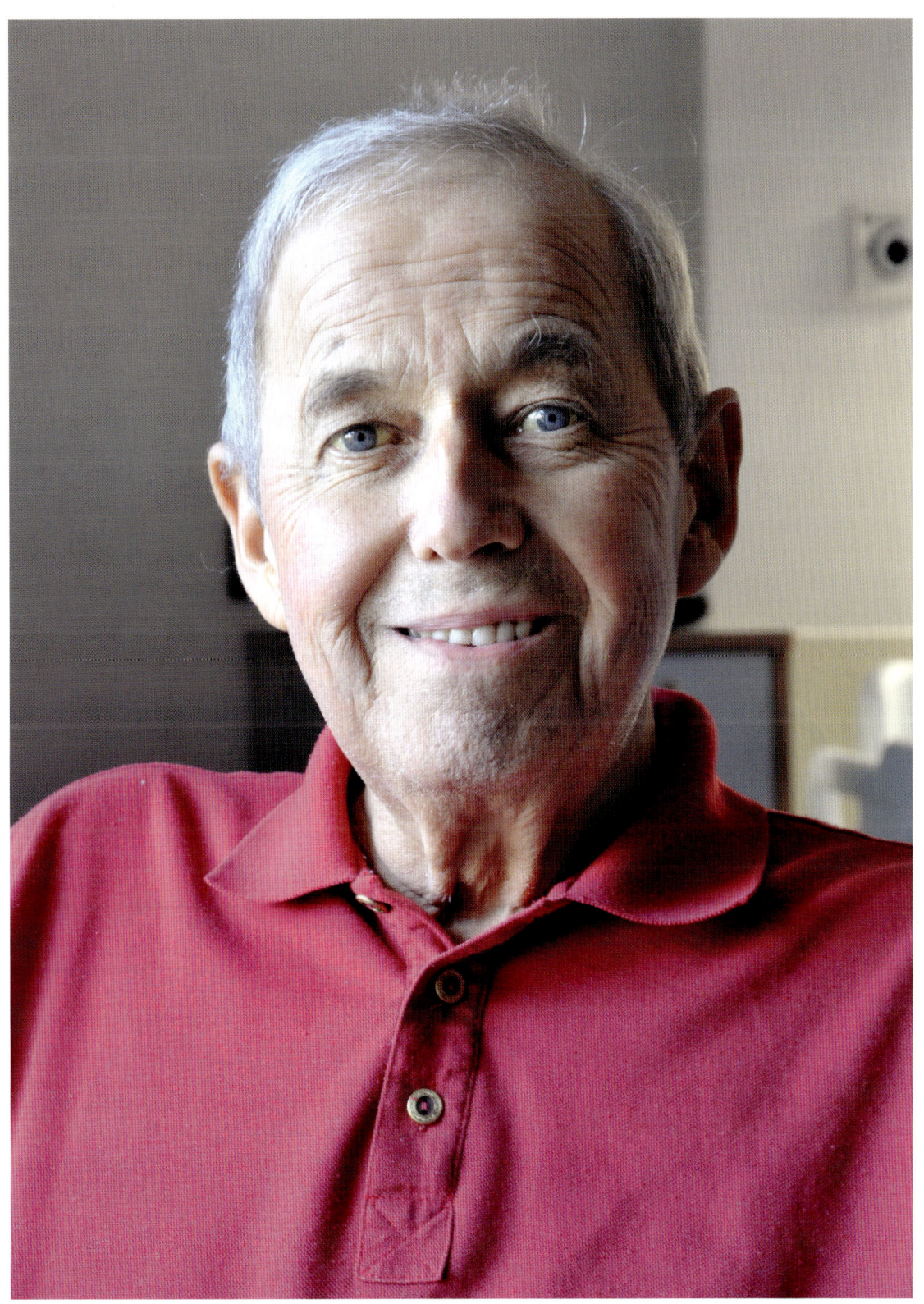

telling me. Apparently, there'd been cancerous cells in my bowel that had spread to the liver. I was almost retired when they told me, so I gave up work after that. I'm 67 now. I'd been driving for Cadbury's and Bulmers for most of my life. I enjoyed my driving job; it was something to do more than anything else. It got me out of the house and I enjoyed it. We took the SAS round the war graves, I enjoyed that. I did a lot of runs to Tenby and Weston-Super-Mare and Aberystwyth. I didn't want to do the ones where I'd be away for a week. I wanted to come home each night. But I did enjoy it. You get a good crowd on the bus, it was alright. The money wasn't up to much but it was a bit of pocket money. But when they diagnosed me, I told them I'd finish. I was having chemo every other week and I knew I wasn't up to it. The chemo knocked me about.

Although I lost my wife a long time ago, I'm not on my own. I've got a son and a daughter, as well. My daughter lives and works in Liverpool so it's more difficult for her to get to see me. But my son's local, he lives and works nearby, so he comes to see me at the hospice all the time. My daughter can't keep going back and forth, she doesn't drive so she'd have to be on the train. It's awkward for her so I told her not to do that.

Things have picked up since I've been at the hospice, they really have. This place is super and I don't know how I'd manage without it. I'm 100% different to how I was a month ago.

It was quite a story how I ended up here. I'd said to my boy: 'Ian, you'll have to get somebody to help me at home', because I knew I wasn't going to make it if I'd have stayed at home. I couldn't get down the stairs, I couldn't get about. Almost the same day, I had a visit from a nurse called Jo, from Macmillan. I must have been on their books, I must have been referred to them. It was as though she somehow knew that I needed help. She told me to get my pyjamas and get a bag and they'd have me at the hospice within the hour. I'm so glad I came here. They really care. It's wrong that it all has to be run on the charity, really. They are spending billions of pounds going to the moon and wasting money on complete rubbish, yet we have to sponsor things like this with charity. It upsets me, it does. It gets to me.

'They are spending billions going to the moon and wasting money on complete rubbish, yet we have to sponsor things like this hospice with charity. It upsets me, it does. It gets to me.'

I'd done my best to struggle on at home before coming here. I'd had some help and they had tried to adapt the place to make it easier for me. They put some handles on the stairs, but it wasn't enough and I didn't feel safe. Now, when I think about it, I know I can't live at home permanently on my own. I can't go down that route because I won't be safe. It would only a matter of time be before I fell. I know I can't make it up and down the stairs in my condition.

While I've been at the hospice, I've had time to think about the future. I don't know what will happen when I get discharged from here but I think I'll have to go to my boy's place, even though he's not got a lot of space. I've got an old three-bedroomed place, it's three-storey house with lots of stairs. It's the opposite of my room here at the hospice, where everything's on one-level and I can wheel myself about with one of those trolley things. I'm fine here. But I wouldn't be able to manage at home.

I did my Will yesterday. The house needs a bit of work doing to it but the kids can sell it at auction and share the money between them. That's the least of my worries. I've got my health to think about and my shoulder is giving me terrible trouble. I just feel absolutely wiped out, you can't describe it. All I feel like doing is sleeping 24/7. I'm absolutely shocked about what's happened, but they have brought me on a lot in the hospice. I know I'm a bloke, but emotionally things can be hard, especially when you have to rely on other people all the time. There are times when things get overpowering.

Being here really lifts my spirits. The room's great. I'd like to get outside because it's a lovely garden there. I might ask my boy to take me out in the car for an hour, just for a change of scene.

My boy told me: 'Dad, we'll take you to the pub'. But I told him no. I laughed. I said: 'The last place I want to go to now is some bloomin' pub'. I think the days of having a pint are over with. The ladies who help out keep coming in and saying: 'Brian, would you like a nice glass of sherry?' It makes me laugh. I say: 'No love, I don't think I should'. There was a time when I'd have drunk a whole bottle. But they are good. They really are. All the helpers and the carers, they do everything they can for you. They're magic.

I knew it was good at St Michael's because of what they did to help my late wife, Mary. We'd been married about 28 years. She got ill when they were treating her for hemorrhoids. She'd be worried because there' be blood in the toilet. My dad would tell me that she looked really ill. I'd tell him that we were back and forth to the doctor and they kept telling us it was hemorrhoids. But it turned out in the end she had cancer.

The tumour was like a bloomin' rugby ball in her stomach. She came here for a few days and they made her better for a while, then she went out. She lasted a little while after but it was no good. She went down quite quickly. My sister was in here, too, and a few of my good friends have been in here.

Obviously, when you're told you can come into the hospice you have mixed feelings. At first I said no because it brought back too many memories. But when they explained how much things had changed, I agreed. At one time, if you came here you only went out one way. And that was in a box. That's what I remembered. So when they asked me it frightened me. But I was wrong about that. They get you better these days. I'm glad I took their advice and came here. I'd thought about going to stay with my brother, Phillip, but I couldn't do that. They've got their lives to lead and they don't need me there.

They've built my appetite up in here as well. Before, I wasn't eating. They gave me some steroids and I built myself up a bit. At home, I'd just be eating a Pot Noodle and that's no good. I was too weak even to make a cup of tea. That was a major effort.

But it's times like this when you need your family. I'm going to get a bed in my son's lounge and I'll be able to manage there. One woman said: 'Do you think you've been a good dad?' And I said I thought I had. They've always had what they've wanted and I've spoiled them if anything; they've had cars, caravans, holidays. Before my daughter went to Liverpool, we had a chat. One of the funny things about her was that she'd never go to the dentist. She's an attractive girl, like. So she decided to go to the dentist before she moved to Liverpool. I told her I'd help her and pay. Then she gave me the bill: £3,500. But you love your kids and you do what you can. You can't say no. She's got a good job and she likes it there and that's all that matters.

My shoulder will improve gradually but it just takes so long. They are working on it and it's getting better. I had a heat bag on it and that helped. The thing is, I want to use it but I can't.

With my liver, I don't know really. I tried to ask the doctor but they don't really know. I asked how long I'd got. I didn't want him to tell me in a way, but I did too. When they diagnosed it in the beginning, the doctor said I'd got 12 months. Well, that's close to three years ago. It knocked me for six when he told me that, I was walking round the lawns of the hospital. But I'm still going.

I didn't know where I was when they told me I'd not got long to live. They sat me down and wanted to have a chat and a cup of tea. I said 'no, just leave me alone, I need to get my head round this'. I had to let the family know, too, which is difficult. They told me as casually as saying 'it's going to rain in an hour'. But that's their job. It's like me telling you how long it takes to drive to Liverpool. They do it every day, so they just get on with it.

You don't really get your head around that stuff, when you're told you're going to die. I didn't believe it when they told me. And then I felt so well for a long time anyway, until I did my shoulder. I just felt so well. But you don't want to believe that you're going to die, that's the last thing you want to hear.

I'm grateful that I've had a long time to live since then and I've had some good times. I took my grandson on holiday to the caravan and had a lovely time. But I know I'm not well, it's just a steady thing that gets worse.

For a while, it looked as though they might be able to help with the liver. We were looking at a transplant, but that idea didn't work out. Then they spoke to a professor at Oxford and he was practicing some new treatment. They asked if I was prepared to go to Oxford to see whether they could try it and I answered: 'I'd be prepared to go to the other side of the world'.

I went down there and he examined me and by the time I got back home, I had a phone call saying it wouldn't work because I wasn't strong enough. So that was a blow. They were having to fly the drugs in from Canada. But I'd just done my shoulder on the Monday and I had the appointment on the Friday.

I'm not surprised they turned me down; all my arm and my side was black from the bruising. I looked as though I was going to keel over in the surgery. If I'd have been well, they might have had a go. I was on Warfarin as well at the time and with that stuff you only have to touch your skin and it bruises. You get a black blister under the skin. When I showed them, they said 'flipping 'eck'. There was bruising all the way down my side, it was solid black. I think that didn't help. My boy said he could see the way the doctor was looking at me and he was thinking: 'No, this isn't going to happen'. And of course I didn't feel well because I'd been in hospital all week. I think the professor looked at me and thought: 'You might as well go back home mate'. I can laugh about it now but at the time it was disappointing. Mind you, it would only have been a trial so there'd have been no guarantees.

I'm hoping I can pick up and go on as long as I can, you know. Everybody tells me I don't look so bad so I'm hoping there's plenty of life left in me yet. They told me three years ago I'd got 12 months; well, I've done okay so far. People tell you different things. Sometimes you think you've got a week, sometimes you think you've got 10.

It's funny the way what people say can play on

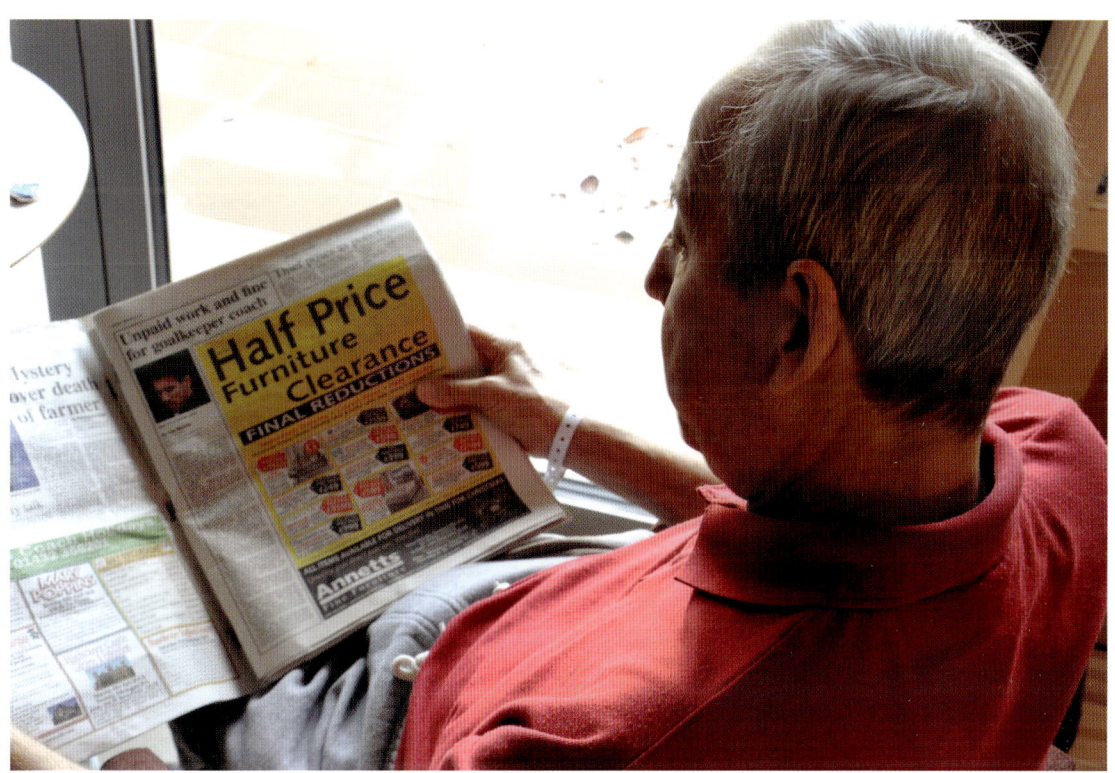

your mind. You know, I've had different doctors telling me different things. I've done my Will now, so that's off my mind and I can relax about things. Being worried is no good, if you're worried it only makes you stressed and that makes you ill. I just make the best of life, to be honest. I try not to read too many things into what people say and just keep going.

I feel alright, my appetite is alright and I don't have too much pain. I'm looking forward to getting out. I just keep going the best I can.

Ethel Evans, 86 The College, Hereford

I've been here two weeks and they've been marvellous. I've got no fault at all. I couldn't get my breath, that's why I came here. I couldn't get my breath at all, but now I can. They've done a wonderful job with me, I feel much better than I did.

I've been poorly on and off for a couple of years. I'd been into the County Hospital in Hereford ever so many times, it's sure to be seven or eight times. That's all over the past two years. It's always been the same thing. We don't really know what it is, it's something to do with my breathing. But I've got heart trouble as well and I've had that for a long time too.

I'm a Forester originally, I'm from the Forest of Dean, but I've been in Hereford for 60 or 65 years. My family were all brought up here. I was 86 last month.

To be truthful I had to go to work because I lost my husband; he died of cancer, and I had four little boys to bring up. I worked at the hospitals, mainly, doing domestic work. I was at the General Hospital for a while.

My husband's name was Vincent White. He was 50 when he passed away and so I had to bring up the four boys. The one boy has since died, that was eight years ago. He had a disease that he caught off the cattle. But the other three boys are all fine. They are all doing very well. They are very regular when it comes to visiting me at the hospice.

My husband and I had been married for a long time. After he died, I remarried and my second husband has been a very good stepdad to the boys. His name is John, but we always call him David. He doesn't like the name John, so we call him David instead. I know that sounds funny.

I retired when I was 60 but John went on working for some time; he worked at a factory down at Rotherwas, Atlas Floors.

I've had a happy life and one of my favourite things was reading. That was always my main hobby. I can't read so much any more because I can't see, I'm partially blind. I can't hear very well either, I'm afraid. It's funny. Never mind, we'll plod on. I'm a happy lady and I make the best of it. And I'm not going to start grumbling now. You have to get on.

Since I've been in the hospice, things have picked up. I don't really know exactly what they've done but it's worked. I came into the hospice by ambulance. I came here for an assessment but they kept me here, they wouldn't let me go back home. I had to stop so that I could get better. I don't mind because it feels worth it. It is well worth it. You learn as you go along. Hopefully, I'll have a bit more treatment, then I'll be home in a few days. So you keep your fingers crossed.

They've given me tablets and a bit of exercise, which has helped considerably. Sometimes I get a little bit out of breath but I'm much better than I was. I feel younger and fitter and healthier.

The nurses are great because they really do care. I wouldn't be here today, I know I wouldn't, if it hadn't have been for the people in this place. Before I came into the hospice, my health was bad. But the people here have been a Godsend.

I'm looking forward to being back home with David, my husband. He's extremely good in the house. I have no grumbles there at all. He's been able to visit me as well. He comes twice a day. I don't know what I'd have done without him. And the boys are very good as well. They come as often as they can. The one boy comes every night. He brings David in because my husband

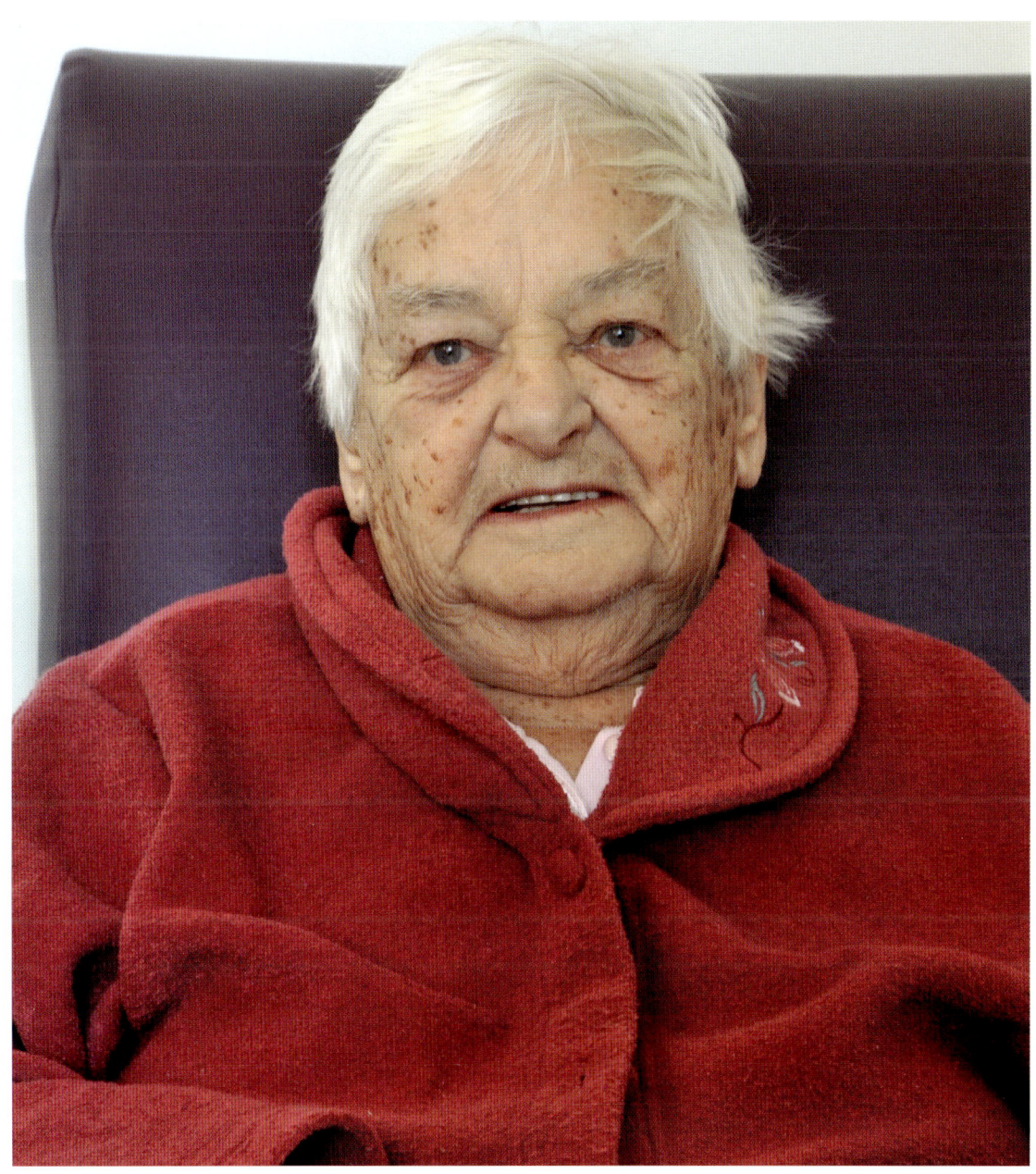

can't drive very much. He brings him down. I've got grandchildren as well. I've got five of them, four great-grandchildren and one great-great grandchild. The great-great grandchild is 12-months-old nearly. His name is Hendrix. It's rather a funny name. He's the fifth generation.

I am very proud. We are hoping to have our photograph taken. We want to get the family together and then we'll see how it goes. My family makes me happy. They give me a lot of joy. I like being altogether. That makes a difference. It's lovely when we're together with the children.

Jade Marie Evans, 20
Chepstow

By Angie, Ed and Ad Evans, Jade's mother, father and youngest brother.

Angie: There were five of us, me and Ed, then Bradley, who's 21, Jade, who was 20, and Ad, who's 14. Jade was poorly throughout her life but she was a great fighter. She was rushed into hospital recently, to Hereford Hospital, because they thought she had a blockage, or some sort of constipation. They did a CT scan but it turned out she had a strangulated bowel. So they operated on Jade that day, it was September 21, 2015, but unfortunately, while the operation went well, she remained very poorly and spent a week in ITU.

We'd spent our lives looking after her. She'd been born at 23 weeks, so she had a lot of problems. Her birth weight had been 1lbs 14oz. She spent most of her time in and out of hospital, particularly when she was younger. She spent three or four months in intensive care.

Ed: From the age of 0-15, there were eight or nine operations. She had a shunt to remove spinal fluid from the head. She had an issue with feeding, she had epilepsy, asthma and blindness. She was a poorly young woman. There were problems with the spine and she had to have an operation to straighten that, using rods.

Angie: She had cerebral palsy as well. She couldn't walk. It was quite hard on the family but we got through it and she kept us going. Her smile kept us pushing forward, as well as the love she gave us.

Ed: She couldn't really communicate well. But we knew when she was upset or when she was happy; 98% of the time it was either smiles or giggles. Everybody else that came into contact with her, people at school, nurses and therapists, they all felt the same; she was a ray of light for everyone.

Angie: Her happiness kept us on track. She'd light up the room. It was difficult, of course, because there was also two other children, Ad, 14, and Bradley, 21. The love they gave her and the love she gave them back was inspirational.

Ad: Obviously, I grew up knowing about her needs. It was confusing at first but as I grew older I understood it better. My older brother understood it well. Jade was a big part of our family. I'd help prepare things for mum, when she was caring for Jade. It was a normal family life. She could let us know she was happy.

Angie: Jade was always in and out of hospital, with chest infections and whatever. She would get through things. It didn't matter what was wrong with her, she'd always come back. She was stubborn and determined. She had operation after operation and was determined to get through. The last one, unfortunately, she just couldn't fight it back. She spent eight weeks and one day in Hereford General. Then we were told about St Michael's Hospice. We really had to fight to get here but we are glad we made it. She came in on the Monday and the hospice people were absolutely fantastic. The care here is amazing. The nurses all fell in love with Jade when they saw her.

Jade was awake on the Monday when we came here, then she fell into a sleep which got deeper, and deeper and deeper. Then on the Saturday morning, me and my husband were washing Jade and we put clean clothes on her. Then when we were changing her sheets and pulling her up the bed, her heart stopped and she passed away. She died peacefully, she still had that happy smile

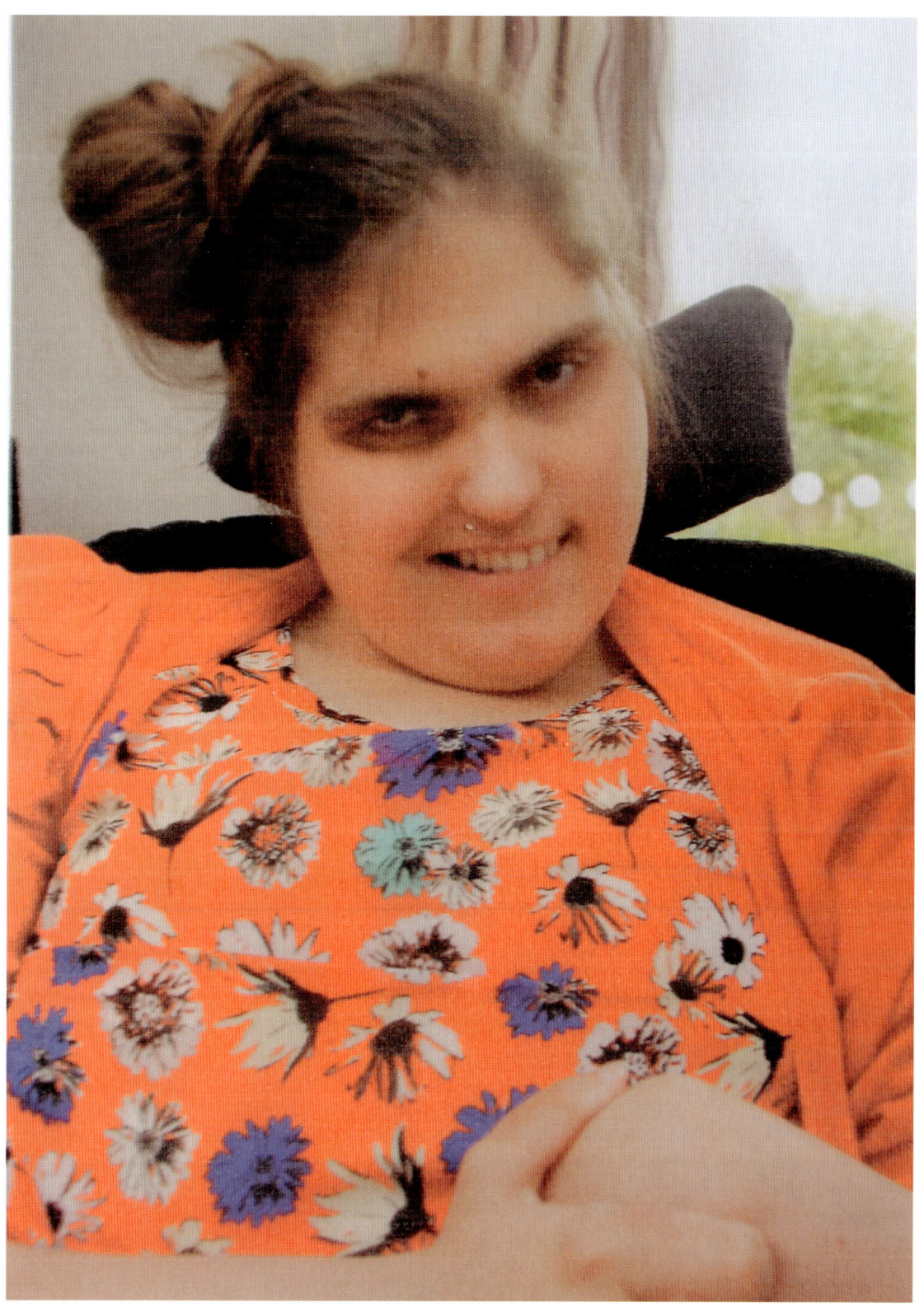

on her face when she passed. I can't thank the staff enough at St Michael's. The doctors, the therapists, the nurses, they were amazing.

Ed: The whole team were remarkable. They were totally consummate professionals from the off. We couldn't fault their work. The way they treat people and look after them is incredible. It's not like a factory where they're in and out. They invest in the people here, whether they are short term or long term. It's totally broadened my horizons. A lot of the patients improve while they are here and then they go home after. It's an incredible environment and the services are remarkable.

From the off, the staff would be honest with us. They talked to us about pain relief to make her comfortable. We could come and go as freely as we wanted to. On most nights, we'd be sat up all night with her. Nothing was too much trouble. It was an end-of-life plan when we came here. Her stomach and bowel wouldn't accept any food, so we were at the end state. There was nowhere else to go. We knew things were coming to the end.

Angie: It was crucial to us that things were good because we'd been crushed like sardines in the hospital. The hospice is more personal, it's a family environment.

Ad: It's like a hotel, almost, for the visitors, with en suite, TV and beds.

Ed: The nurses respected people's feelings and our privacy. It was a home from home. We were able to care for our beautiful daughter. It was time to say goodbye but we could do that with dignity and peacefully.

Angie: We had Jade's funeral and we asked for donations to St Michael's Hospice. That's what Jade would have wanted.

Ed: There's no funding for this, so it's important to us that people understand the need to fund it.

Angie: It meant the world to us to have time with Jade, that last week. We spent as much quality time as we could and that meant so much to us as a family.

Ed: The doctors and nurses were able to do what they needed to, but we had that time which was the most precious and important thing of all.

Angie: I had my doubts about a hospice. It felt like a black cloud over my head. I'd heard about them and was worried. But we were told by the hospital to come and have a look so that we could see what we thought. So we did, we came here and it completely opened my eyes. I fell in love with it straight away. It was the best thing that could have happened, it was the best thing for Jade.

You have to remember Jade was a loving and lovely girl. She'd get frustrated with certain music. If a sad song was playing she'd get unhappy and would start biting her finger to let us know. If Adam came in and was in trouble and her dad's voice would rise, she'd start laughing. She had a wicked sense of humour. She loved the announcements in the shops, the one that say:

'The whole team were remarkable. They were totally consummate professionals from the off. The way they treat people and look after them is incredible.'

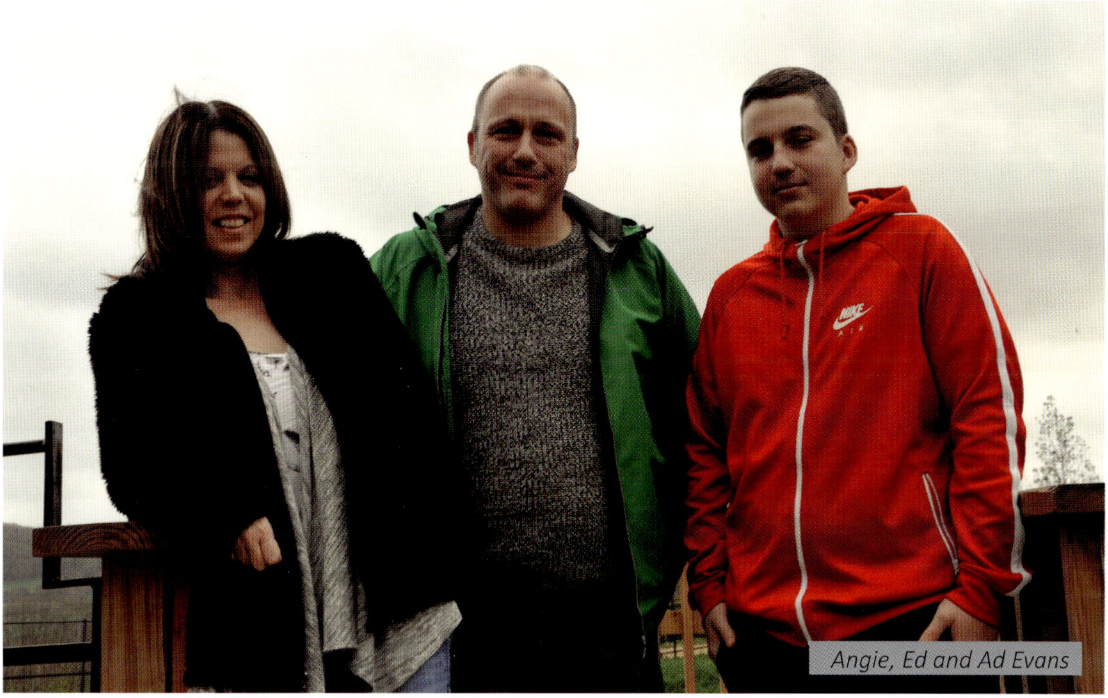

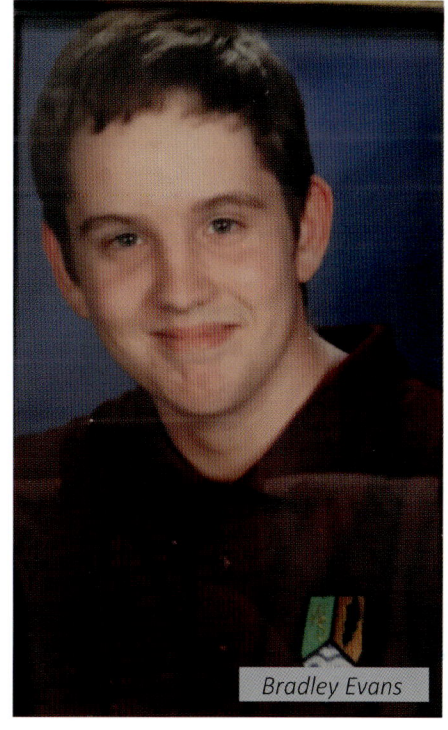

Angie, Ed and Ad Evans

'Cashier Number three, please'. She'd giggle her head off. If we were in TK Maxx, she'd just be laughing at the announcements. If people were in her way, she'd kick them. She did a sly boot. She couldn't see them but she could sense them. She used to be very, very cheeky. It was just that smile. No matter what she went through, how poorly she was, she'd just smile and light up the room.

Ed: She was always listening. Her hearing must have been so sensitive. Her eyes would flicker to wherever the sounds were.

Ad: If somebody coughed, she'd be looking straight away. Or if someone sneezed, she'd have a giggle fit.

Angie: She was such a happy girl. She loved her music, she loved her hydrotherapy and her rebound on the trampoline. But she hated her physiotherapy, she didn't like that. Her arms were

Bradley Evans

quite tight because of the cerebral palsy. She didn't want to know.

Ed: She had a major operation on her back and we thought we were going to lose her then. She'd have been about 14 and the operation was in two stages.

Angie: The operation was eight hours and the next operation was 10-and-a-half. She was very unpredictable then, on the second part of the operation. But she needed it done because her spine was crushing her lungs. Afterwards, she was still smiling.

Ed: She'd have a day or two when she was a bit groggy and then she'd smile.

Angie: It helped us so much to know she was so happy.

Ed: Jade was a poorly girl so at first it was a big learning curve. We tried to treat her like a normal baby but things would go wrong, like she wouldn't take a bottle. It was a learning curve over the years to understand what was happening to her body and how she was coping with it. We got to learn things over time.

Angie: The doctors were straight with us and told us Jade would be lucky if she made it to 16. She made it past 16 and got to 20. I just wanted to be a bit greedy and have her with us for a little bit longer.

Ed: She battled well all the way through her life, to 20. We're so proud of her.

Angie: I was with her every day. She made the most of things. My husband was in the Army and was away in Afghanistan. I must admit, Jade was the one who kept me going, just with her smile and being happy. She brought us so much love and happiness. I do miss her.

Ed: All the teachers and therapists who met her bonded with her quickly. She had such personality. She also knew how much we loved her. She'd recognise our voices or she'd put her hand on our faces to feel for stubble or a nose.

Ad: She'd put her hand next to me, or rub my head.

Ed: If there was someone she wasn't sure of, she'd bat them away or throw a teddy bear at them. She had her ways. She was a beautiful young woman.

Angie: She'd love going in the car over the speed bumps. She'd laugh.

Ed: I'd be driving the car and I'd tell her. I'd say: 'Way up', and she'd laugh as we went over a bump, then 'Way down', on our way back down. She just laughed and laughed and laughed.

Angie: When it came to the end, the hospice were amazing.

Ed: They've all been totally compassionate and they've got their own sense of humour. They've been trained so well and are so accustomed to these things. They made us feel at ease. A lot of people might be put off because of the stress of dying, but they don't. They just know how things are.

Angie: They've been absolutely fantastic. I'm just grateful we got our daughter here in time. We loved her with all our hearts and this was the best place for us to say goodbye to her.

By Bradley Evans

Where to start?

Jade was born 22nd April 1995 at Darlington Memorial Hospital. She was the middle sibling of the famliy.

Jade had her medical disabilities but in my eyes that made her the person she was: warm, gentle and full of life.

Wherever you would go she would always have a smile so bright it was hard not to be infected by it. She gave people enormous joy.

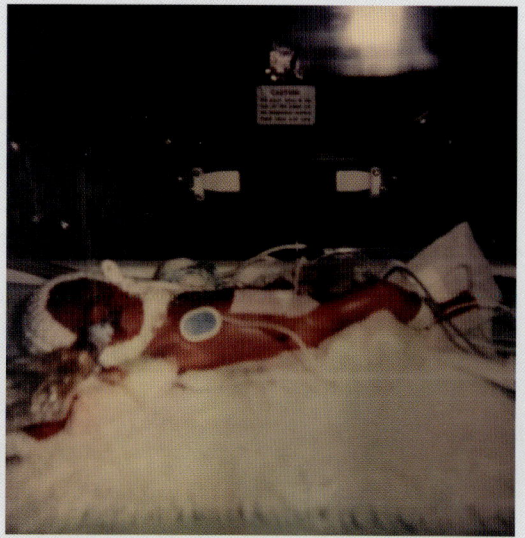

No matter how much pain she was in, she would always smile. Jade was and still is the stitches that hold our family together. Even now, after her passing, she binds us more tightly than ever.

Even though Jade has started a journey to some other place, I know that the joy and happiness she brought me and others will never fade. The best way to describe Jade is by using the words that were on her casket: 'A smile to inspire'.

That's exactly what she had and I wouldn't be half the man I am today if she hadn't been brought into this world.

She had a smile so bright and a laugh so sweet. They are now gone but will never be forgotten.

Janet Griffin, 74 Rhayader

Let me start by saying the most important thing: I haven't come here to die. That's the thing that everybody gets wrong when they hear that you're in a hospice. When you say the word 'hospice' people actually hear the word 'death'. Well I've not come here to die. I've come here to get better. I'm going to go home and carry on living.

I've no plans to die in the hospice, although, when the time comes to say goodbye, perhaps I'll change my mind and come back here because the people at St Michael's have been so remarkable during my stay.

I first become poorly 12 years ago. The cancer came in my breast in 2003 and I went to Abergavenny and Cardiff for the treatment. I went through the whole process, from beginning to end, and in 2009 they told me I was clear. Then the cancer came back in 2012, in the liver. Soon after that, it went into my bones. So I've been having treatment ever since, at Hereford Hospital. I initially went to the doctor, then I came to Hereford Hospital. So I've been very, very lucky up until now.

The cancer causes a lot of pain. I've had some radiotherapy on my hip, which helped to clear it up for a while. But it's come back with a vengeance and I'm walking with sticks.

At the moment, because of the pain, my oncologist doesn't want me to go down the chemotherapy route. He wants to get the pain under control before looking at treatment options and that's why I'm here, that's been my route to the hospice.

The pain, well, what can I say? There's no routine. Every time something happens you lose a bit more. At first, I was walking with one stick but then it got so bad that I could hardly walk at all and I had to have two sticks. That dragged me right down emotionally. I had to deal with the pain as well as the loss of independence. My independence and mobility were severely compromised. I went down mentally, too, I had had enough. That phase lasted for three weeks. We live in a very rural area, so we're quite isolated, and after three weeks I'd had enough.

I live with my husband, who is a little older than me. He's 86 and not in very good health himself. I've always been the driver in our relationship, so when I couldn't get around I got very down. I was very low, very, very, very low, as though I'd had enough. I felt: 'what else will happen?'

As part of my treatment, the Macmillan nurses came on the scene. They tried one or two different pain killers but in the end they decided to send me here so that they could get the pain under control and monitor me. If I'm at home they can't do that. The treatment that I've been having has helped, it's certainly helped.

So far, I've been here nine days and I'm going home tomorrow. I think, if I stay here much longer I'll lose more of my independence so I'm keen to get home. The hospice has given me respite and I know that if I get to another low ebb and need to come back then I'll be able to, it's no problem.

The staff understand how the patients feel; that's one of the good things about St Michael's. I'm a people person, I like other people. So being here, in a friendly environment, helps to remove the issues of isolation that there were when I was marooned at home. It's like someone's thrown a switch and I'm back to my old self. I'm back. I can cope again. I went off track because I'd had enough. But this is it now, I'm back on track.

I can combine visits here with being at home. I can come to the day centre, too, once I've gone back home. Even though it's an hour-and-a-half away, they will pick me up and bring me here. So I can live at home but stay on track with the hospice.

I've felt very comfortable here, too. My room is lovely and there's a beautiful garden outside too. It doesn't compare to the views at home; when I look out of my window there I just see rolling countryisde. There's the most wonderful bird feeder, too. I can sit in the conservatory and watch the birds all day. But it's been brilliant here too, it really has.

When I first came in I had young Dr Hazel. Well, my daughter couldn't get over the way she was talking to me straight away. She had such empathy and understanding. She was absolutely lovely. The fact that there are people like that gives everyone a lift. My daughter, for instance, was over the moon, as were my friends, because I found a doctor who understood. I found somebody who was determined to do something to help me. I'm not being left to struggle on. With Macmillan nurses, they can call in and stay for half an hour, but that's all they have time for. They are too busy to stay. But here, they are for you. They are with you.

The peace and tranquillity of St Michael's helps, too. It's very tranquil. I sleep so well. I wake up lying there, thinking 'this is lovely'. If I'd been at home, I wouldn't have the pain under control. It's been brilliant, honestly.

Before I came here, I was struggling. My friend came to visit me and I could scarcely walk to the door. I had absolutely had enough. I'd been like that for a couple of weeks. I still get pain now, but it's more manageable. The cancer is in my joints,

so when I walk the pressure creates pain. If I'm sitting or standing still, I'm fine. But I don't want to spend my life sitting or standing still. I take medication to alleviate the pain. I can get up and get about, to a certain extent. It's much better. I don't want to sit and vegetate. Everything's improved. They have definitely helped me.

There are a couple of aspects to being poorly. There's the physical effects, obviously, but there's also the way it makes you feel. They sort of go hand in hand. Now that the pain's stable, I am looking better and getting my spirits back. All of my friends say that, even the staff do.

I wouldn't hesitate to recommend people going to a hospice. When people know you are going, they are a bit shocked. The word 'hospice' frightens people. They think you're going to die. They think that's the end. But I knew that was wrong even before I came here. My daughter went on line for me and she knew that it was a place where you can start to get better. She came off her computer and said: 'Oh mum, they do all sorts of things there'. And I said: 'Yes, I know they do'. I've had quite a few visitors, it's a home-from-home.

The level of respite is amazing, too. My husband and I have both been ill, so it's been hard for us. I've been in charge and looking after him but with me going down a bit it's been a bit fraught. Hopefully, when I go back, we'll be fine. We do things together and we get by. We've got a smallholding, that's the trouble. We've got five-and-a-half acres. We let the fields to the neighbours, so they look after them. But there are still a lot of general things to do like the garden,

> 'Being here helps remove the issues of isolation that there were when I was marooned at home.'

which my husband does. We've lived there for 15 years.

We bought the smallholding for when we retired, which was 2000. I'd had a few health issues, including a pelvic floor repair. I'm a tall lady and I used to work at a nursing home for people with MS. In those days, we did all the lifting ourselves. We did it physically and because of my size I used to take a lot on. When patients were on the floor behind the door, people would come and fetch me to lift them: 'Jan, can you help'. I always did. I was 59 when I left the care home. My husband has always been a country lad and my daughter was out in Wales, so we wanted to get back to the country.

Before that, I'd done all sorts of things. When I first left school I went on the market gardens because I wanted to work on the land. I had a winter of riding my bike down the Kenilworth road to a nursery. I went and worked there for 12 months. But after one winter of that: no! I went to work at Marks & Spencer. And I stopped there until I had my child. After that, I became a dinner lady, then I had a job in the corner shop. I started working as an ambulance driver in an old people's home when I was 40 and I worked on the wards too as an auxiliary. Working at Helen Ley was where I was happiest. There was something about that place that was really special. Everybody got on really well and we all loved the patients. I took to it like a duck to water, it was absolutely fantastic. I loved every minute of it. I was there nearly 20 years. Socially and professionally, it was great. Once I'd left the care home, I kept in touch with my friends and a few of

us are still together. There's a bond between us. We've all stuck together, through the years. Now I need my team, I need my friends around me.

I think I've done well not to have to use the hospice before, if I'm being honest. When I had the last lot of cancer in 2012, they gave me 12-18 months to live. I should have been gone at least 18 months ago, or more. But I'm still here. We still haven't worked out a route map, but I know I've improved. I think we'll be going down the chemotherapy road again when I get out.

There's a lot of fear when you're ill. And what the hospice also does is give you a safety net. Emotionally and physically, the hospice gives me a break. It's respite but it's more than that. If I found myself struggling at home and needed a place when they were full, I know they'd put me on a waiting list. They're the light at the end of the tunnel. I know there's something that can be done. And when you feel happier, you also feel healthier. That's one of the things that St Michael's gives me. It's as though they've flicked the switch, I feel as though they've found the switch and got me going again. I feel better mentally and as though I'm more in control. That gives me the strength to cope with the pain and with everything else that's going on. If the pain defeats you and makes you miserable, then it's harder to cope. When the pain is at the front of everything, you feel defeated. But when you feel mentally strong, the pain doesn't feel so bad.

When you get cancer, you're in a fight. Everybody is concerned about you and wants to know how you are, but the truth is that they want you to tell them that you're fine. They don't want

> '**There's a lot of fear when you're ill. And what the hospice also does is give you a safety net.**'

you to be: 'Oh no, I've got to go and have this done and that done, I'm not very well'. People don't really want to hear that because they lead busy lives. They want you to tell them that you're fine. If you tell them that you're doing alright or that you're amazing, then it makes them feel happy. You can almost hear them go: 'phew'. Because then they don't have to worry. One of my friends will say: 'How can you be ill, your voice is so strong?' And I say: 'Well what do you want my voice to be like? I'm just talking. The cancer's in my liver and bones, not my voice'.

You put on a brave face for your family and friends. If they're not sure, they might not ring because they don't want any bad news. It's easier to just tell people: 'I'm very well'. The 'cancer' word frightens people. We all know cancer's not contagious but some people treat it as though it is. It's almost taboo. People don't want to use the word 'cancer' because it frightens them. It's the same misconception that people have with hospice. They think hospices are all about dying, but they're not. And they think cancer means you're going to die, but it can be beaten.

I realised I was ill this time around during a night out. I was going down to Leamington to stop with my friend and see my brother and have a nice time. It was a break, retail therapy with the girls. There was a party at where we used to work and I went down to that, at Helen Ley Care Centre. I had a pain in my side, I didn't know whether it was indigestion or what it was. I didn't say anything about it and the pain went to a certain extent, but not altogether. When I got home, I went to see my GP. My doctor told me

he'd send me for an ultrasound scan. I went for that and then my husband and I were called in to say there were cancerous cysts on the liver. I went from there. I was absolutely fuming. I was so mad and cross. Because why? Why again? I've had it once. I've been down that road. I've done all the things. And there it was again. It took me a little while to get my head around it. Perhaps I'm still like that. Perhaps that's why I am the way I am. That's perhaps why I'm so positive about it.

My husband said: 'How long?' And the doctor said I'd got 12/18 months. He said it wasn't operable because it was in the liver and also because it was lots of little nodules and cysts, rather than a tumour. So we went down the chemo road, then down the Herceptin road, and I've been fine.

When you're ill, one of the things you want most of all is to be treated normally. And this place has been brilliant. It's my first taste of a hospice and it's done the trick. It's been better than my expectations. There have been all sorts of complementary treatments and there's a day centre too.

I think because of my background in a nursing home, I had a good idea of what it would be like. But I didn't realise it would be as good as it has been. On the first day I was here, the nurses offered to wash my back. Well, I could have cried.

Actually, I did because I'd been unable to wash my back. It was absolutely amazing. The nurse dried it and then dried my feet. And it was incredible because those are things I'd been unable to do. But from then on, Miss Independent has done everything herself because they've got enough to do without fussing after me. I'm just focused on getting better.

'When you're ill, one of the things you want most of all is to be treated normally.'

It might seem silly, but I feel as though I'm lucky to have had all this extra time. They told me 12/18 months and I'm still going strong. But at the back of your mind you also know that the extra time will stop at some point. Eventually, you'll go along and the doctor will say he can't do anything more. I'm geared up for that and I just enjoy each day. I just think I'm lucky. I'd rather be healthy, of course, and able to do everything that I used to do. You give up a lot because of being poorly. But I just think of myself as being lucky. I've got to make the best of my life. That's what I think. I have to try my best to master it and make the best of it. My friends and family are with me; those bonds are never broken.

I think my background in nursing helps me to understand this better. I certainly get good vibes from being here. At Helen Ley, they used to say there was an aura and there is here too. The building is right in the countryside, with an apple orchard and hills. I was talking to my stepson last night and he was in France. He said there's a wonderful full moon outside my window. And I looked out of my window and it was there, too.

'But I just think of myself as being lucky. I've got to make the best of my life. That's what I think. I have to try my best to master it and make the best of it. My friends and family are with me; those bonds are never broken.'

Cicely and Cyril Bownes, 82 & 83 Shobdon

Cyril: I lived in Ludlow all my life, before moving out to Shobdon 18 months ago.

Cicely: I lived in Steventon. I was there from the age of two. But these days I find myself at the hospice and I seem to have been here forever. I say that because it feels like home. The staff here are so good to us.

Cyril: It's about three or four weeks, I think. They've been marvellous.

Cicely: I have cancer in my lung, that's why I'm here. I was in Hereford Hospital and it was more or less decided that I would come here instead. They are very pleased with things, so am I. I had a chest infection three weeks ago and couldn't breathe. I just felt thoroughly poorly, now I'm pleased with life again.

Cyril: She's pleased with life. She's improving all the time.

Cicely: My legs had given up on me but they're coming back. I'm happy and the nurses are happy with my progress too. The people here care, very much so.

Cyril: They improve things here that they can't do in the hospital.

Cicely: At hospitals, they have too many patients and not enough staff. Here they are just so wonderful. They are kindness itself. They never come through the door without a smile on their face and I'm sure they don't always feel like smiling. But they always come through with a smile. They are truly wonderful.

Cyril: It's a wonderful place.

Cicely: When my husband wants to come and stay for the day, they're marvellous about it. They don't hestitate. They tell him to order a dinner from the chef. There's no argument at all. It is marvellous.

Cyril: It's great. Cicely gets plenty of visitors.

Cicely: Our eldest son Cyril brought him in this morning and our eldest granddaughter will pick him up on the way home tonight, so we get to spend the day together. We started with two sons, then we grew a little bit to three granddaughters and three grandsons, now we've grown a little more to six great grandsons and two great grandsons. I did tell the eldest granddaughter that I'm waiting for the next generation. But she told me not to wait for her. They can all come here. The girls live around Shobdon and Pembridge and one or other of them come every day. The family come when they can. I tell them not to worry, I tell them just to come when they can. My great grandsons come, the eldest is 20, then 18, then 14.

Cyril: We've lived happy lives. I was a self-employed electrician in Ludlow and had a business for 40 years. But I've been retired for 20 odd years.

Cicely: Our retirement life has been good. We didn't do all we intended doing, you never do.

Cyril: You make a list of places you want to go to but you don't cross many off. For a few years we had a static caravan on the Welsh coast that we used and enjoyed. The kids used and enjoyed that too. It was between Barmouth and Harlech.

Cicely: The main thing we have is each other. We have been together for 66 years. We got together through a friend of mine. I was taken on a blind date, unknown to me. I met him and that was that. It went from there. The blind date was in Lower Gladeford. My friend had to go in an evening to collect a jug of cider. In those days, there were little off licences and there'd be a wooden door inside. You'll collect beer or cider

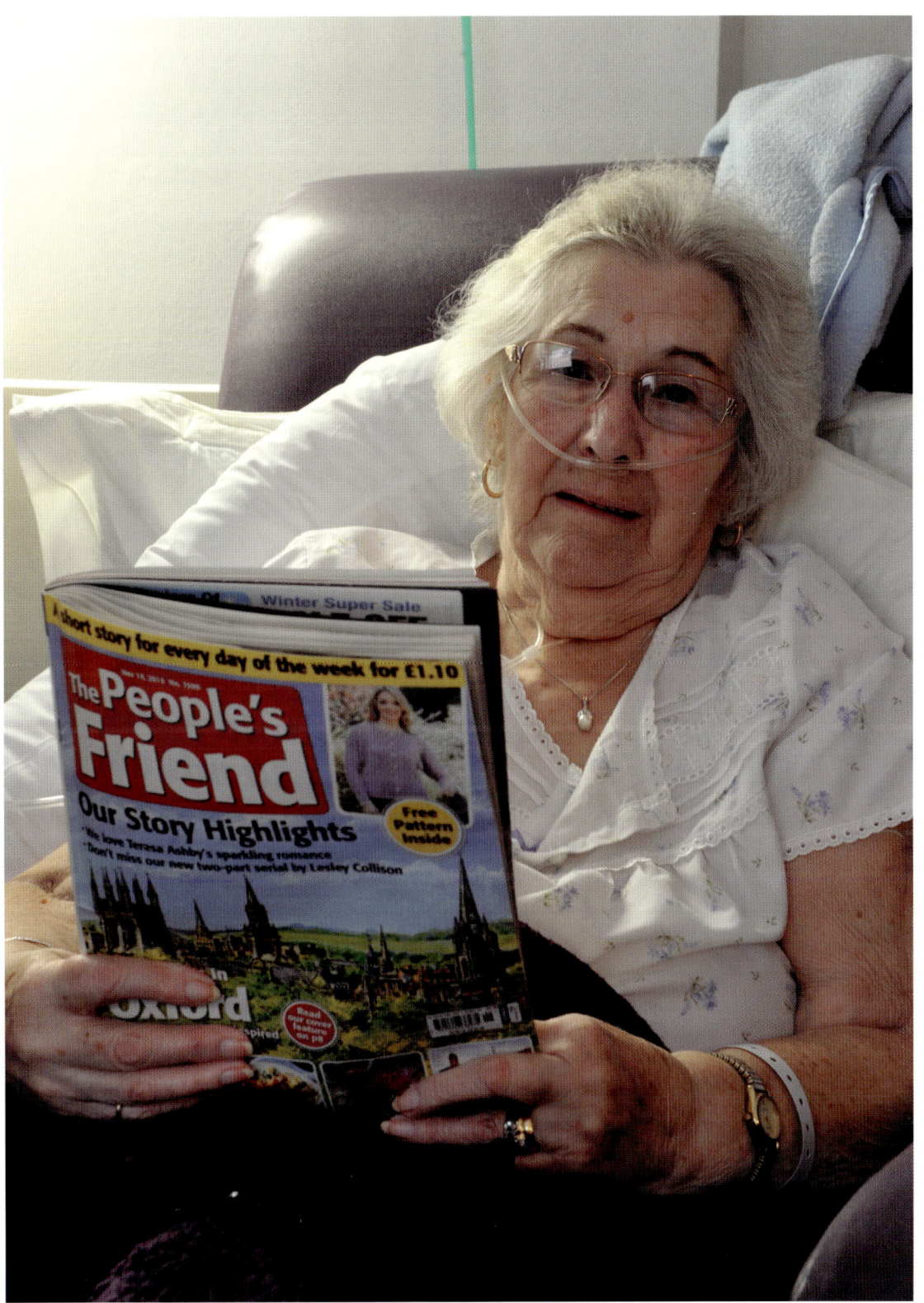

there. My friend's father always wanted a jug of cider, so she'd go there. One night, she told me to go with her. I had nothing else to do. It turned out she was meeting a boyfriend and he'd taken Cyril with him. The rest was history. I was 15 and Cyril was 16.

Cyril: We were together for a couple of years then got married. We went to the registry office.

Cicely: My father told me we were too young. I told him we were not. Both sets of parents were very supportive.

Cyril: I served an apprenticeship, four years part time at Shrewsbury Tech. And then I started on my own. I had up to three guys working for me and some were on a casual basis.

Cicely: Then I would look after the children at home. Unfortunately, I started having heart attacks when I was quite young. I had the first one when I was 38. I started spending quite a lot of time in Shrewsbury Hospital. I've had four altogether. They were coronary thrombosis, which is a clot going through the heart. Unfortunately, two of them didn't go through; they went halfway and decided to stop, which was a bit of a menace. It was a long, long time before I had the next one. I thought they'd forgotten about me.

Cyril: Then we both had strokes. We went through a spell of clear weather before then. But then we had our strokes.

Cicely: I had five altogether, but we weathered them and saw them off. They weren't too serious. They just affected my right leg and right arm, but the movement has come back more or less.

Cyril: But we've always been here for one another. We've worked hard. We had a shop selling electrical stuff in Ludlow for a while as well as my electrical business.

Cicely: You know, we consider ourselves fortunate. We've had good lives, happy lives. And I still consider myself fortunate. I am lucky to be at the hospice. If it wasn't for the hospice I don't think I would be here today. Their kindness is

remarkable. I can't describe it. It doesn't matter what time of the night I ring for them, they come and they are smiling. Nothing is too much trouble for them. When I came here first, I was dubious about ringing the bell. I would wait and wait and wait. Then I would realise it was no good and that I needed their help. So I would call them and they would really get cross with me for not calling sooner. But now, I still don't ring it for every triviality but they are so helpful. They are committed and devoted. There is real dedication, it's nothing to do with wages.

It lifts the mood being here, which makes me feel happier and healthier. After a couple of days in here I felt that I wanted to be out of bed. Whereas before, I was quite content to lie in bed. After two days, I wanted to help and not let them do everything for me. They are just so kind.

Cyril: She has made very good progress since she's been here. She now manages to walk with her frame. Before, she couldn't pick her leg up.

Cicely: Everything is better since being here. I am forever grateful.

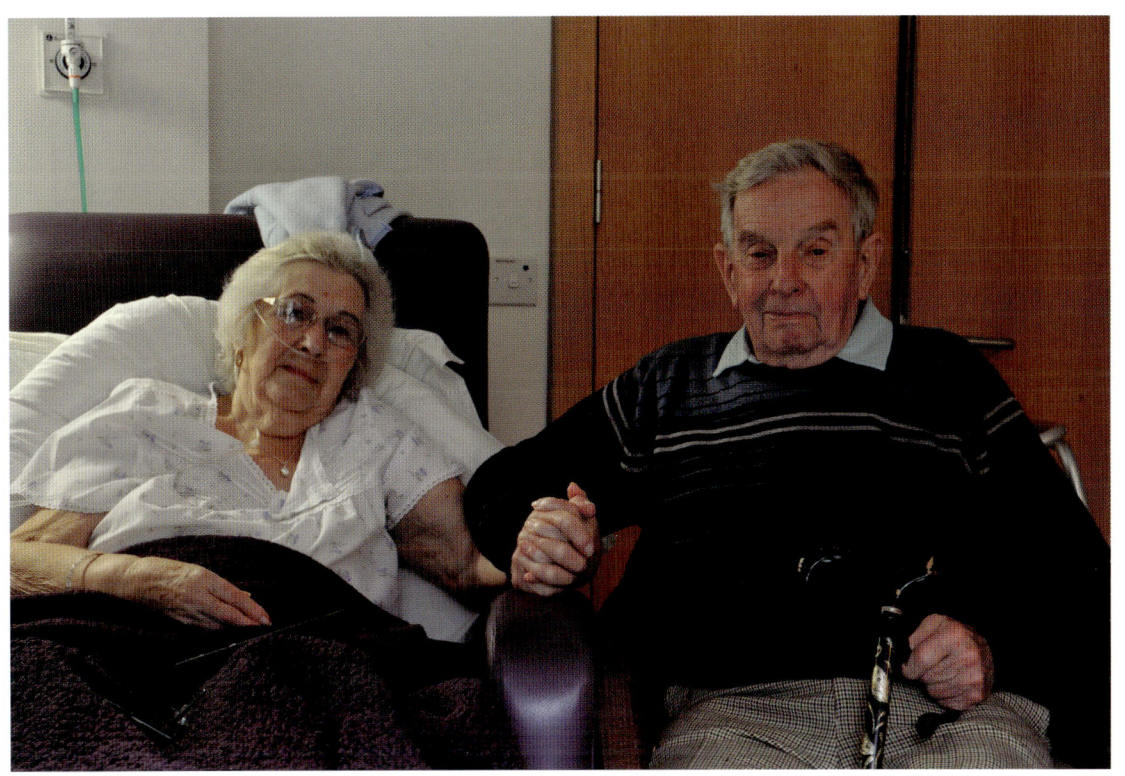

'Their kindness is remarkable.
I can't describe it. It doesn't
matter what time of the night
I ring for them, they come and
they are smiling. Nothing is
too much trouble for them.'

Pam Beeby, 62
Weobley

In December 2006 I was diagnosed with colorectal cancer. So for a whole year, from December 2006 to December 2007, I was in and out of here constantly.

If I wasn't in hospital, I'd be here. The tumour was sitting on my coccyx, so it made it impossible for me to sit down at all, so I was at home on my own and couldn't leave the house. I had to either stand or lie down. So I spent a lot of time in here. I couldn't go out because the only way I could leave the house was in an ambulance and on a stretcher. So I got quite run down and depressed and had panic attacks. If they had vacancies here, they would ring me up and I'd come in. That was the first time I'd been very poorly.

In the January I had an exploratory operation and in the February I had a colostomy and they decided that the tumour was very large and they didn't know whether they could operate or not. After that I had a massive infection and I came in here and I was in here for a couple of months until they had sorted it out and I was in a fit state to go home. It was just amazing. I don't know what I would have done without them.

I was acutely depressed. My husband had passed away about three years before so I was living on my own and living very rurally. Although my family and three children were around me, I was alone. I was still grieving my husband in addition to fighting the effects of illness. So I would come here for the day in an ambulance and then they would say they had a space and they'd let me stay for a week or a fortnight. Or I'd go into hospital and then be transferred here.

I was never resistant to coming into the hospice. It was me that asked. I had the colostomy in Hereford Hospital and spent eight days in there: I wasn't given a bath, I wasn't looked at, I wasn't fed properly. By the time I came in here, the infection was so bad that the first thing they did was bath me and clean up the wound. They had to send for a surgeon from the hospital to come and take all the stitches out and then they had to put a vacuum dressing on it to draw out all of the fluid. I was in a terrible state and it was purely from neglect. I think at that point, I was here for a couple of months. My mental state then was poor; I wasn't at all happy. So it helped a lot to have people around who cared and were professional. At that point, I had to face the prospect of chemotherapy and radiotherapy. I knew that there was also a massive operation. I had all that in my head and I was also wondering how I would cope with it. The only way I coped with it was because I was receiving help from here. On a practical level, I needed help. I needed carers at home for the periods I was at home. I was also physically sick, so I couldn't eat and became very thin and very weak. So I had no energy to do anything. I got to the point where I could get out of bed and walk to the end of the bed and that was the furthest I could go.

After the first operation, in the February, I had a period where I recovered here from the operation and infection. Then I went home for a period and they wanted me to go straight into Cheltenham Hospital to have chemotherapy and radiotherapy together because the tumour was so vigorous and large. If they hadn't reduced it down there would have been no chance of them reducing it and no chance of me surviving.

So I went home and tried to build myself up physically and mentally. I did pick up a little bit. And then in the May I went into Cheltenham Hospital, I was still quite poorly at that point and wasn't able to do anything at home. I had

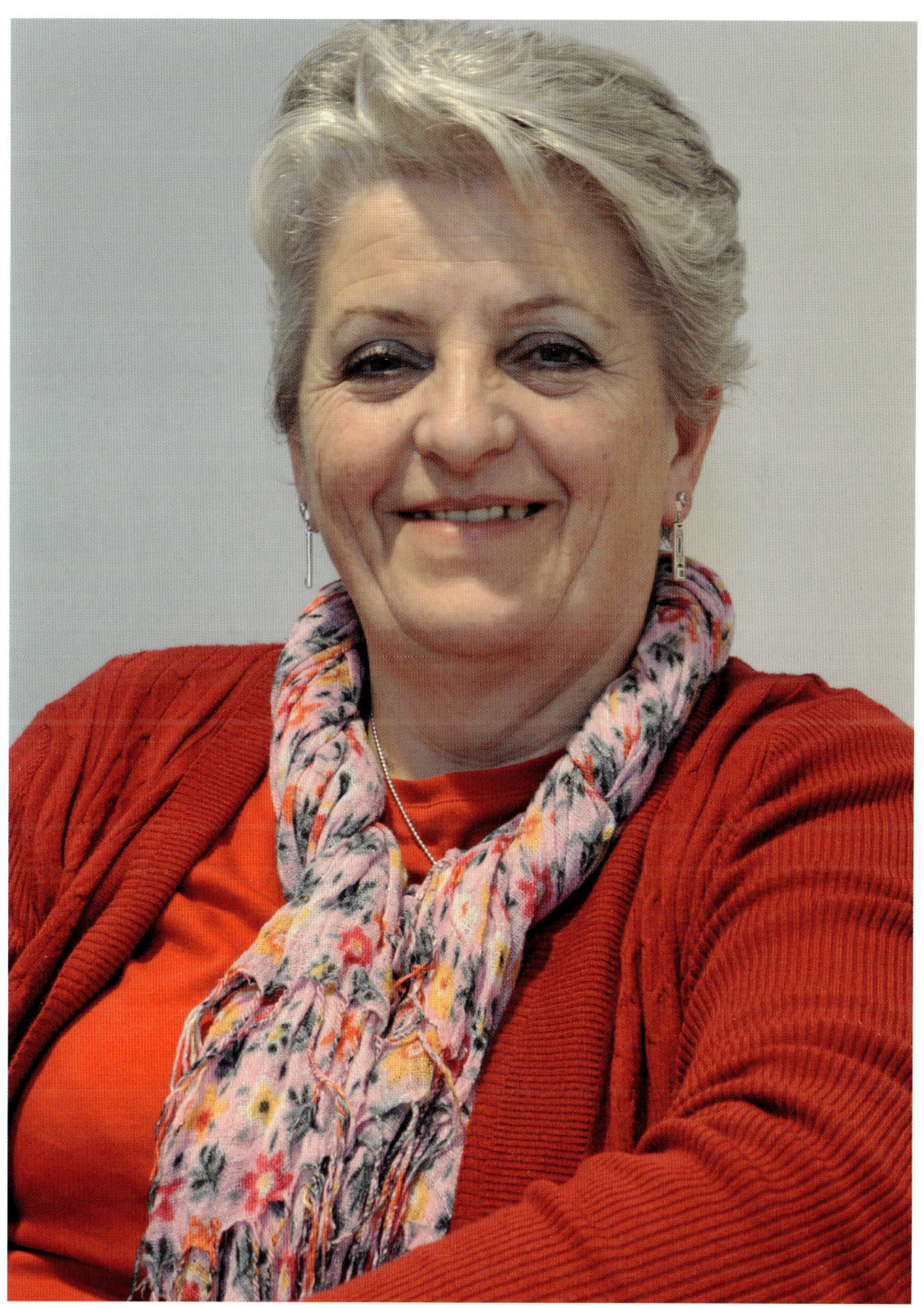

people in most of the time. They started the chemotherapy and radiotherapy and I stayed in Cheltenham for six weeks. When I came out, it had shrunk the tumour down quite considerably. So that was good news. But then I had to wait to build myself up again because I knew in myself I was too poorly to then go and have major surgery. The surgery was going to be really intrusive. So I came to the hospice again. But on and off, all the time, I was getting infections. I got cellulitis in my legs a couple of times, which made me really ill. I'd maybe go into the hospital a couple of days and then I'd come here, I'd end up being in here for ages. My daughter used to say that when I was in the hospice, she could go home and go to sleep. But she'd say when I was in the hospital, she'd just be thinking about how to get me out of there.

You know, just being able to do the simple things here meant the world to me; like being able to have a bath, or relax, or do nice things. I couldn't do that at the hospital but at the hospice there would be somebody there. If I was at home, I would be spending all of my time on my own. I would have Macmillan Nurses, but that was only for a short time. So I would worry about falling, I would have panic attacks. I was afraid of everything because I literally couldn't do anything. I could only walk from my bed to the bathroom and I spent too long on my own. The last carer would maybe come at 7pm or 10pm and I would be on my own for 12 hours. The only thing I had was a telephone. At that point we were having lots of storms. If the electricity had gone off, I wouldn't have had a phone or a light or anything. I was panicking. I had candles

everywhere, matches everywhere, just in case something happened. It was very isolating, it was awful. And I was still grieving for my husband.

My mood gradually improved. I would have reflexology, aromatherapy, counselling and other services when I came to the hospice. I would have music therapy, too. I remember the first time I was wheeled in from the ambulance. It took less than 24 hours to get me into the ward. When they wheeled me into the hospice there was a lady sitting in the corner playing a harp. It was so lovely and peaceful. The whole atmosphere was totally and utterly different. When you feel happier, it helps you physically. You start to believe you can cope. But to do it on your own is impossible.

I eventually had an operation to remove the tumour. But the tumour was so large and so close to the coccyx that they said they couldn't remove the tumour unless they also removed the coccyx. It would have been pointless because it was a vigorous type of cancer. So I went in and they attempted to operate but they weren't able to do it. The tumour had grown back and become too large again. So I was sent home and I came back in here again. My daughter went to see the surgeon and asked if there was anybody else in the country who could do the operation. She said there were surgeons in Leeds and London who might be able to help. So the surgeon in Leeds told me he could do it but it would be massive surgery. It was October 19 2007 when I underwent surgery. I was in Leeds for three weeks afterwards and I couldn't keep any fluids down at all. They removed my rectum and a lot of the soft tissue. I was cut all the way down my back, with bone removed.

'You know, just being able to do the simple things here meant the world to me'

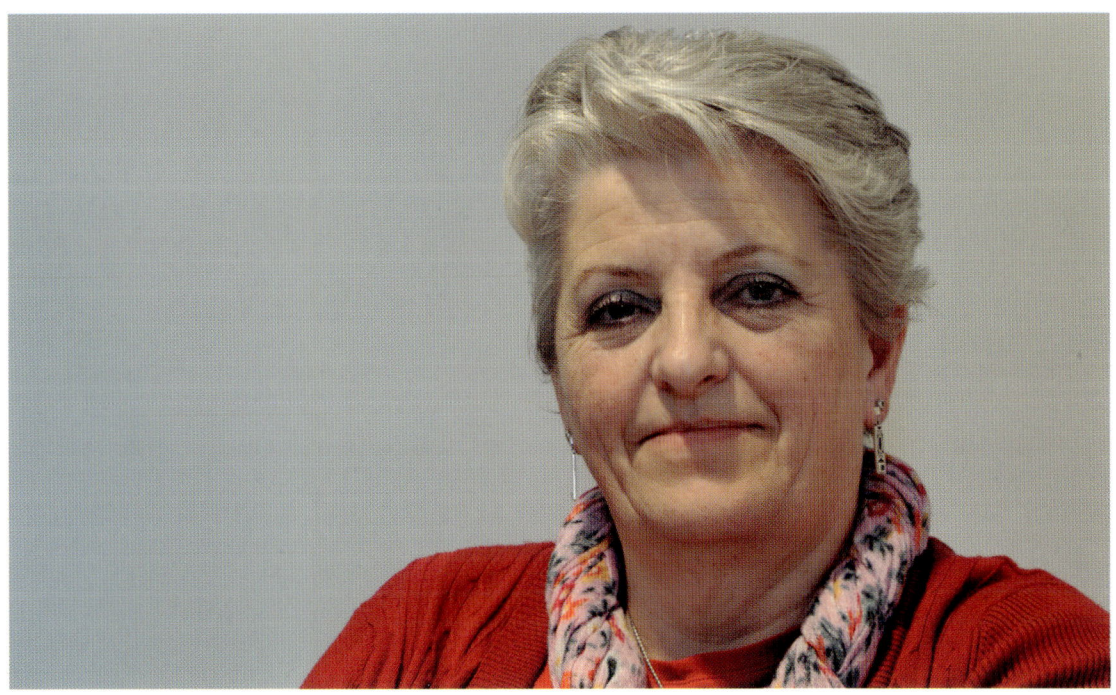

I had about 10 days at home and was really struggling. I'd also got so thin. So I spent a week in here to try and see if they could stop me being sick. Then I ended up having to go back into hospital where I was tube-fed for five weeks to try to get my stomach used to being fed again.

They managed to take the tumour away but I now have problems because I can't walk very well or sit very well. So there were huge consequences of the surgery. It saved my life but there was a price to pay. I have to cope with pain on a day-to-day basis and that's been since October 2007. So I still come back here for a day, for the Living Well clinic. I have severe neuropathic pain because so much soft tissue has been taken away, the nerves branch off like trees and each of those nerve endings is painful. The whole of my rear is quite uncomfortable. I can't stand or walk for very long and I can't sit for very long. I have to keep moving all the time and I still don't have a great amount of energy. But the support I get from here is amazing.

Basically, I had to learn to walk again. It took me two years to get back on my feet and learn how to drive a car again. Up until then, I was improving. But then that improvement stopped. I realised a long time ago that this is how it's going to be. It's not going to improve. The way I am now is the way I'll always be. But I have ongoing help from St Michael's.

There are other challenges, of course. I lost my son-in-law in April 2012. He was in and out of here. He was a Peruvian guy who was married to my middle daughter. So we've had a lot of support since that. There's been help in terms of grieving and counselling. It was a help to the whole family, we had the help when he was in here and after he passed away there was the opportunity to reflect. The hospice really helped to lift our spirits. I've had a year of counselling for everything, really, which has been amazing. It's really helped. It's given me new ways to look at things, new ways to cope.

I can look at situations and cope much better. I can cope better with people if they upset me or stress me out, for instance. It's been a really tough decade. Losing my husband was the first thing and that genuinely knocked me for six. I had cancer, I lost both my parents within the space of six months and then my daughter lost her husband. It's like having the rug pulled completely from underneath you and you get to the stage where you wonder what else can go wrong.

Without being able to come here and sit and talk with people, I don't know what I'd have done. When my parents died, for instance, there were difficulties within our family. I was affected a great deal by the things that happened. Trying to cope with all that was remarkably difficult and I received cognitive therapy, which helped. They gave me new ways to connect and cope. I've found different ways of doing things, which has helped me to come to terms with everything that's happened.

Cognitive therapy was particularly good. I would spend an hour with someone and look at different ways of coping. It's made me so much stronger. I can be more assertive. My attitude has changed.

The work that the staff do here is just amazing. It's like coming into a family where everybody wants to help. I can't stress how important that is because there would be days otherwise where you'd want to jump off a cliff. They can help. They can get things done much more quickly than if you just went to a GP. There's always somebody here. They have a movie night once a month, which is really nice. You can come and get together with other people who have problems.

It's everything to know that you're not alone. However bad it gets, you always know there's somebody else there. You also get perspective and strength. You know that there are other people who are worse off. If you are feeling low or fed up, you look at others and count your blessings. It's invaluable really.

My daughter and son-in-law have raised money for the hospice. We try to give back when we are able to. We can't always do that, but we do our best. We are eternally grateful for everything St Michael's has done for us.

My daughter and son-in-law have raised money for the hospice. We try to give back when we are able to. We can't always do that, but we do our best. We are eternally grateful for everything St Michael's has done for us.'

Terry Knight, 76 Hereford

I was diagnosed with cancer of the liver in April 2015. It was most unusual. I was working out in Holmer gym and would go there three times a week. I was as fit as a fiddle.

Overnight, I just turned yellow. It was very, very noticeable. I rang up my GP and he told me to see him straight away. They told me I had jaundice, though they didn't understand why. They decided to take me down to the hospital for scans. I had four scans of varying intensity and they couldn't find the source. They knew that my bile duct was blocked and therefore the bile was not reaching my stomach, liver and kidneys to do the work it should do, with the result of the yellow colour.

I stayed in hospital overnight and had a full body scan, which took an hour-and-a-half. Then the consultant came in during the afternoon, sat on my bed and told me they had found the source. He told me I had cancer of the liver. It had killed off one complete side of the liver. That was it. Out they went. It's quite frightening to be told that when you're on your own and expecting the results of a scan for jaundice. To say you become shellshocked is not quite correct. But what did happen was that everything seemed to go over my head. I felt as though everything wasn't happening to me. Just before the consultant left, I asked him for my prognosis. He told me I would have about a year to live, though it might be two. I'm presently halfway through my first year.

Since then, the treatment I've had has been unbelievable, it's been absolutely fantastic. I refused chemotherapy and radiotherapy because I want to maintain my quality of life. I don't want to be bald and I don't want to be in a wheelchair. I don't want to go through so many negative processes in order to extend my life by an extra three-to-six months. I want to be lucid and I want to enjoy what I have. I've told everybody, I've not hidden it. I told my family, who were devastated at first, of course. And their support and the support of my friends is quite unbelievable. What I would say is that it has taught me that there is a big ignorance about cancer. There are so many myths and I find that you've got to be quite dominant and assertive with others. You have to say to people: 'look, I might look ravaged on the outside, I might have lost two-and-a-half stone, but inside, I'm me. I'm still looking at you as I was. Let's carry on as we were'. That's what I say. You see, I don't want sympathy. I don't want gushing love. I just want to carry on and do what I can within my fitness regime.

I didn't talk things over with anybody. I just felt that this would be the best way I could handle it. I get grey days. I get blue days when the world comes crashing down on me. Then I sit quietly and read a book. That's the way I handle it. My wife now has realised that if I'm in a grey area, she just needs to let me go and not fuss over me. I don't want another cup of tea. I just need to carry on as we were. I might have days where I'm not too good, but then I know that the next day I might get out in the garden. I don't sleep well anymore and haven't for a while. They gave me sleeping pills but I became a zombie the next day. It was hilarious. I just kept falling asleep.

I've always been an active man. I didn't have a degree after school, though I found I enjoyed instructing others. I ended up as Assistant County Commissioner for the Scout Association. I would train new leaders and young adults. I loved it. One day somebody told me that I was good at helping others and I ought to think about teaching. There was a course, a Certificate of Education

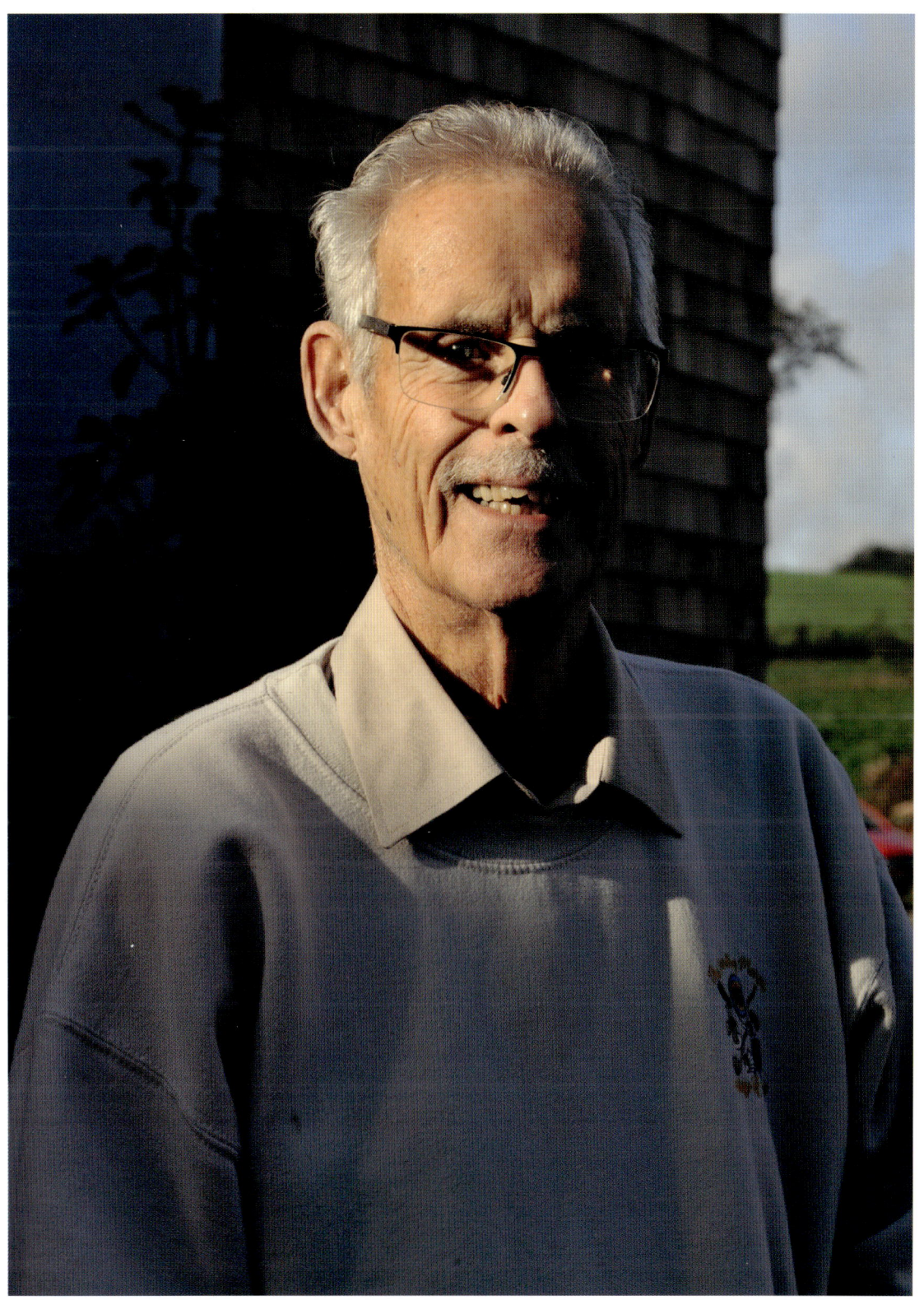

that I could take, which I took and passed. I liked it. Then I was encouraged to build on that. I found out about the Open University and over a number of years I got a BA in history and English. Then I did a BSC (Hons) in criminology and environmental science. Then I decided to go one step further and get a PGCE. So from being a self-appointed, sort of not-very-clever guy, who was just average, I managed to extend my ability. In a period of time, I really did become well qualified, which led to better jobs. It was very much a voyage of self-discovery. I never thought of it as being a sacrifice. There was always something different around the corner. The people with degrees got there with hard work, so I just thought I ought to give it a try. There was no feeling of wanting to show off. I just wanted to be me and see how far I could go. I spent eight years in education and I was asked if I wanted to carry on and do my masters, but by then I was a little burned out. But I felt 10 feet tall when I graduated and had my photograph taken with a mortar board. It was so fantastic for me to be able to say to myself: 'I'm part of this, I'm here with them, not watching them'. I did it to prove something to myself. My father had taken me out of school early, you see. I proved that maybe he was wrong because I achieved something. I would have been in my 30s at the time. It was a good experience. If I can do it, others can. I'm nothing special. I don't like people who moan about their lot in life; I think they should go and do it.

I've always enjoyed trying to give something back to the community and in addition to my leadership work with the scouts I was also with the St John Ambulance. I was the County Staff Officer there. I was a trainer there again. I loved

'I loved bringing the best out of people.'

that. They gave me a service medal with the order of St John, which was quite pleasing. I retired when I was nudging 70 to let others take over.

I loved bringing the best out of people. This is the part of life that somehow society seems to have lost. This notion of care and empowerment, this desire to bring on potential by encouraging and guiding and training is so important. It doesn't matter if people achieve a low mark or a high, what matters is that people do the best they can. I loved being part of that process, of putting the groundwork in. You train, encourage and then let go. I didn't do it for any rewards; that would have been a false world. I did it because I thought it was the right thing for me and because it enabled me to help others.

Sport has played a big part in my life, too. The main sport I have loved is flat green bowling, which I've done over many years. I've been very fortunate to play for the President of England's team, which was a nice honour. Then I wanted to learn the laws of the game, so as to better understand it. I then became an umpire. I am still an international umpire. That's another world of etiquette and politeness. It's wonderful being out in the open air and walking up and down, then socialising afterwards. Over the years, it's been a big part of life for both my wife and I. My wife did extremely well and got to national finals. Now, with my illness, I have been weakened to a point where I can't really push those bowls up a heavy green. But I loved the challenge while I was able to do it. I became a coach in that, too. If you were to put me in a box, the biggest one would be training. That has been my forte throughout my life.

In 1977, my love of training was recognised with a British Empire Medal. I was a very proud recipient of that. It's still in the drawer. It was a nice tangible piece of recognition. I accepted it on behalf of all the teams I'd worked with. I received a phonecall asking me whether I would accept it, then I received a letter with the details for the presentation. It was great. I would never wear it. The honours system later changed and I received an MBE.

When I look back at my life and particularly my experience of training, it's easy to draw a number of conclusions. My philosophy on training is that I can widen the knowledge of others and give them more self-respect and confidence. To do that, I constantly remind myself not to take others for granted. People have their own lives. They know their own worth.

In the keep fit world, I've made some lovely friends. One of them had a daughter who took her GCSE mock exams and she did terribly badly in English. Her parents asked me if I'd help her. They told me they'd pay me but I refused. So I took her under my wing and went to her house every Thursday until she took her GCSEs. She got an A. That was my reward. She took her exams and did very well. Her potential came out.

Now, I come here for physiotherapy. I have lost a lot of muscle, which was quite appalling. My Macmillan nurse recommended I come here. When I started, I was as weak as a kitten, which felt terrible after previously being so fit. I am now building my strength up and I enjoy it here. St Michael's is like a tranquil oasis. There is no panic, there is no rushing around like you get in a hospital. You look at the grounds and the fountains and it is peaceful. I could quite happily end my days here, that's what I'd like to do. If I am blue or not feeling too good, I get an immediate feeling of calm when I arrive here. This place is so, so special. I know that the time ahead is not going to be pretty good. I am prepared for that. I have accepted it. But this place, just to come and sit and have a workout and talk – it's absolutely brilliant.

I am realistic. You know, I have a disease and it is going to kill me. It is going to change me, physically, in a way that is undesirable. I don't like this new me, I feel skinny and I was nice and robust. But that is part of growing into a new phase of my life. At 76, I have had lovely experiences. I have reached my levels of attainment and achievement. Nobody can take that away from me. I'm still very active. I meet my old gym buddies, I take part in pub quizzes. I think I realise when people don't want to hear anymore and I stop talking then. I respect people's need for space.

My Macmillan nurse and the staff here play an important part in my life. They have come in and created a lovely caring shield. For instance, I wanted to go back to my old gym and both of them warned me that I wasn't ready. They were right. They have given me a series of exercises instead that I can do at home and in the hospice. You know, until you are in this situation, it's impossible to realise how important St Michael's Hospice is. Society is still terribly ignorant about how cancer affects the whole tenure of your life. The moment you mention cancer, people either go into a sort-of: 'Wow, what do I say now?' phase. Or, they want to go too deep.

St Michael's is a place where people come to live. Yes it might be painful and yes people might slip into a coma towards the end, but that is nature's way of putting people to sleep. You just drift. There is nothing to be frightened of. I have had a good life, I have a good marriage, I have wonderful grandchildren. There is nothing I could recommend more highly than St Michael's Hospice. It has everything you need when there is a major problem. People do not shout at you or bully you. St Michael's is like a pair of arms that just reach out and hold you.

Tessa Huggett, 74 Culmington, South Shropshire

Partner: Ken Hotchkiss, 80, Clee Hill

Tessa: I have MND. The first indication that there was a problem was about two-and-a-half years ago. My partner will answer some of the questions for me but I will also answer them on my light writer because I can no longer talk. We have been partners for 25 years.

Ken: We were in France visiting a friend and Tessa lost her voice for no apparent reason. We thought she had some sort of bug. Her voice completely went. There was quite a lot of leg pulling and banter. Little did we realise that it was very serious. We came back and it got worse and worse. Eventually, my friends at the local golf club and the bridge club encouraged her to see someone. As well as problems with her voice, Tessa was having trouble moving the cards around when she was playing bridge.

Tessa: So I went to see a doctor, but I was very reluctant. I thought I'd had a stroke.

Ken: We went through a series of doctors. There was a throat specialist, then a speech therapist and eventually we got to a neurologist who was 80% sure of what it was but needed a second opinion. He sent her to see the consultant at the Queen Elizabeth in Birmingham. He virtually confirmed it then, but needed further tests. There's no actual test for MND, it's a series of eliminations: once you've eliminated everything else, you're left with that. Over a period of two months, it became obvious what it was.

Tessa: In France, we had gone out to look after a friends' dogs.

Ken: We had a dog-sitting venture that developed over the years. Our friends would ask us to go and look after their dogs, so we'd go all over the country and France to stay in people's homes while they were away. She also took up repairing pottery and that led to a short career as a sort of antiques dealer. In between that, she also played golf. That's how the two of us met. It was 25 years ago. Between dog sitting and antique dealing and playing golf, Tessa was running around everywhere and anywhere for many years.

Tessa: I have always been a very fit and active lady. I was an outdoor physical education teacher. I loved outdoor activities. My main area was up in the Yorkshire Dales.

Ken: Each day, she would take parties of children up and down mountains. There was kayaking and caving and lots of walking. Then there was golf. Tessa would play off 23 and I would play off about eight-10. Wherever we have been to dog sit, we've usually played golf as well. We've found the most gorgeous courses and been welcomed wherever we've played. We've played in Cumbria and Scotland and France.

Tessa: I camped, sailed, dived and did everything.

Ken: She's also dived and swum in both the Antarctic and the Arctic. Tessa's mother was ill, many years ago, and Tessa looked after her. At the end, when her mother died, Tessa decided she must do the things she wanted to do. She wanted to go to do something special and decided to go to the Antarctic, where she'd always wanted to go.

Tessa: At the outdoor pursuits centre where I worked, in Yorkshire, there was a girl called Molly Porter. She had a husband who worked in Antarctica. That helped to inspire me to go.

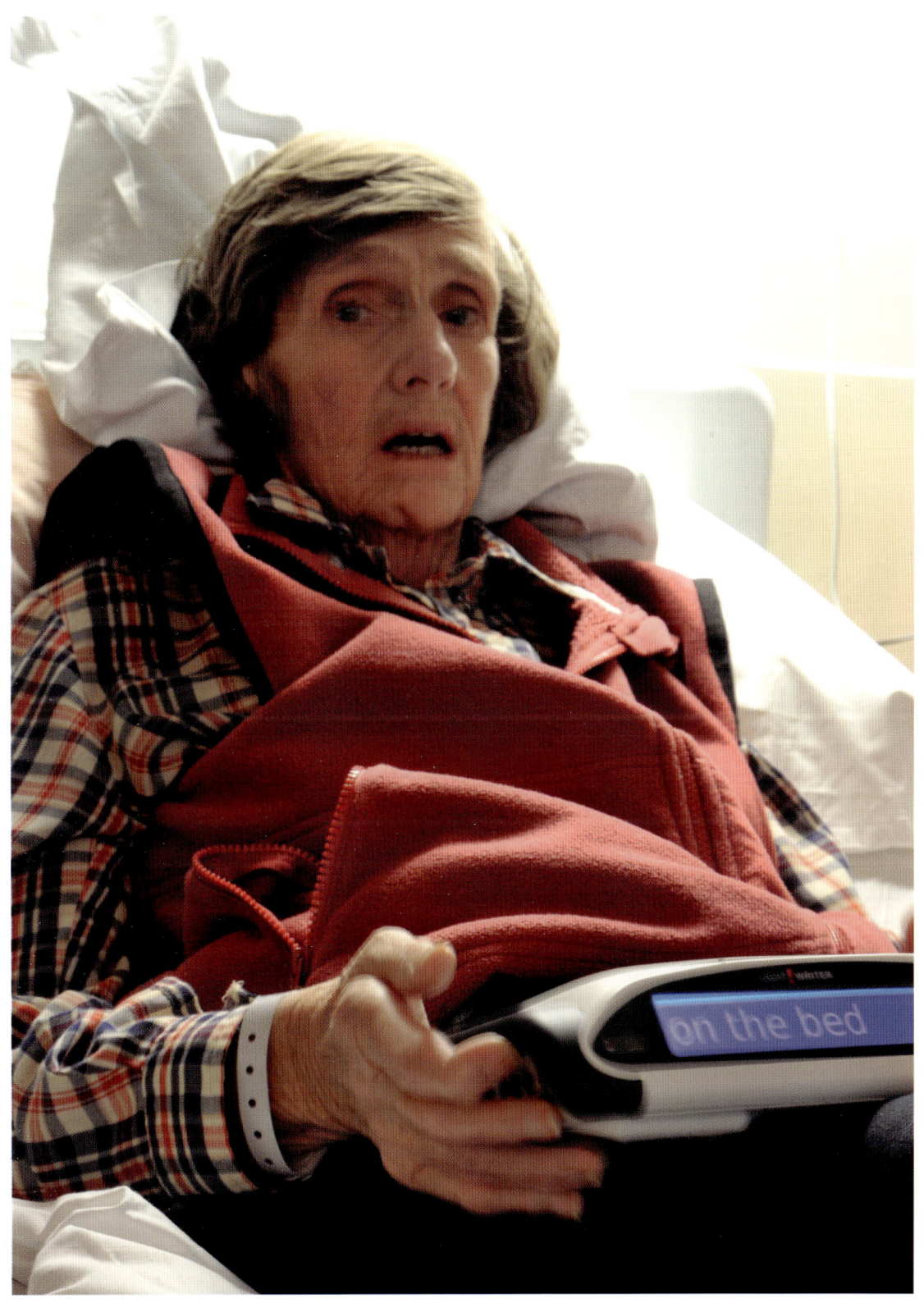

Ken: She has led a remarkably active life and at one stage booked a passage on a boat going round the Antarctic. She went and had a day in Buenos Aires. As a single person, she had to share a cabin and she ended up with a fascinating Australian lady. They hit it off immediately. At the end of the trip to Antarctica, she went to Australia and backpacked all the way up the East Coast and swam on the Great Barrier reef before ending up in Darwin. On the way back home, she stopped off in New Zealand and backpacked all the way along New Zealand.

Tessa: I went to Scott's Base Camp and it was just as they'd left it.

Ken: The Antarctic was always a dream place for Tessa. That's where she'd always wanted to go.

Tessa: I got time off from the outdoor pursuits centre and I raised several thousand pounds. I got it all organised.

Ken: One of the things as part of the cruise was the opportunity to swim in the sea in the Antarctic. Tessa has a certificate to show that she actually swam in the sea, which was signed by the captain of the boat.

Tessa: There was ice climbing, too. We would also go to the Cairngorms, in Scotland, each year.

Ken: You can see the effect of this MND on a person who has been so fit throughout her life. You can see from her various stories how she has been tremendously active throughout her life, from never standing still, to being in a bed. It comes as a desperate shock. We had visited the hospice before, as an outpatient, and the service was tremendous. Little did we realise there was the back-up facilities here. It was only when the hospice care nurses visited that we were introduced to this. The facilities and the care have been second to none. Nobody can question it. It really has been a great help to Tessa. She has been concerned about me having to look after her all the time and putting my own life on hold. So to come in here and be looked after, with expert medical attention, has been an absolute boon. It's been tremendous.

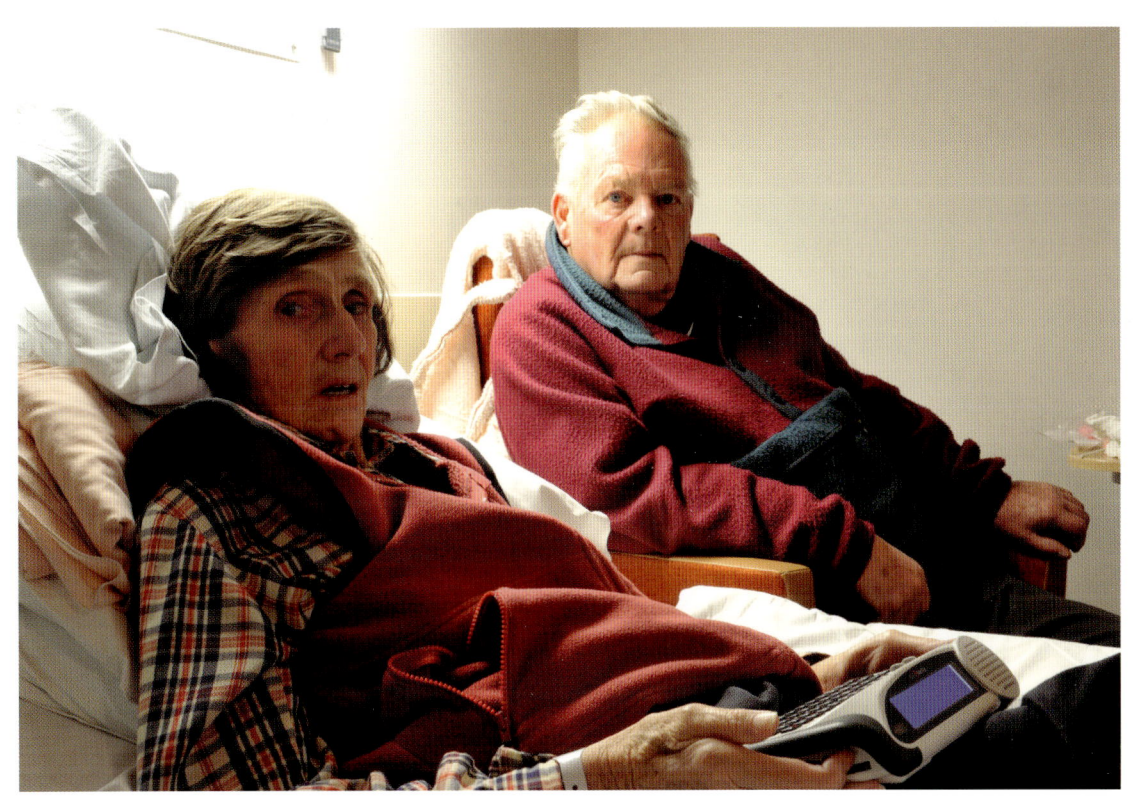

'You can see the effect of this MND on a person who has been so fit throughout her life. You can see from her various stories how she has been tremendously active. It comes as a desperate shock.'

Ann Kay, 72
Woonton,
Herefordshire

've been here for three weeks so far. It's because I have bone metastasis. It's secondary cancer in the bone, which is an extremely painful little thing. I'm not getting well, but hopefully to a situation where I can go home. I had breast cancer, prior to that. The breast cancer has caused the bone metastasis: it went to the bone, that's how I see it. It all started in March/April this year.

I started to get pain, basically. The pain with bone problems is quite nasty, basically. I've probably got a number of broken bones in the spine. It hurts. That's why I spend a lot of time lying down. It's easier than sitting up and supporting your back.

But I don't just want to talk about being ill. That's boring. I'd rather tell you about my life. I started out in the valleys, in South Wales. I was very happy there. I can't think of anything negative to say. I had a happy childhood then went to Swansea University and studied English and History. I didn't do much work, though. I have to say I was a very lazy person. But I did enjoy it. I was going out with a fella from Blackwood when I went to university, but it didn't last. Life was too exciting. I enjoyed being a student very much. It was good fun.

After university, I became a teacher. That hadn't been in my plan: I didn't have a clue what I wanted to do, being honest. In the 1960s, there was very little careers advice. Nowadays, you're inundated with advice, but back then we just made it up as we went along.

I went to Birmingham because my boyfriend at the time was there. He became my first husband. He was a Welshman, his name was David. I was 22. We were together until he died. He went to Aston University and I went to Great Barr Comprehensive School as a teacher. We bought a house near West Bromwich, on a little housing estate called Charlemont. It was near to a motorway and a railway line; it was a nice little house. We were there for seven years and I loved it. After that, we moved to Leicestershire. My husband got a job with Roadstone, Tarmac. I was still teaching, by then I'd discovered that I loved it.

We did okay. We had two cars and a happy life. Teaching was fun, I really really enjoyed it. The kids and me had a laugh. I didn't feel as though I was some sort of guru for them. I just thought I was hanging on by the skin of my teeth. I taught history and I can remember teaching Anglo Saxon. I did English too, and I recall teaching the poetry of Philip Larkin. There were some challenges: at one point I became pregnant but lost the child.

In Leicestershire, I discovered a superb school called Countesthrope College. It was an exceptional school. It was a liberating place. It was a wonderful place for kids to develop. I absolutely loved teaching at that school. I learned such a lot. I learned about democracy. I learned how slow the process is, but how interesting it is. I learned how to empower kids: if you give them stuff they will be empowered. I worked there for almost 30 years. I went there in 1972. My husband died in 1990 and I left there in 2002, something like that.

My husband had motor neurone disease, so he had six years of being ill. It wasn't great.

Then I got married again to my second husband, Jeff Kay. We moved to Kington, in north Herefordshire. Jeff's a headteacher at Kington. We met at Countesthorpe College. We both wanted to move; that was 13 years ago. I was ill with breast cancer and wanted to be nearer to my father, who was in south Wales. It's very unusual

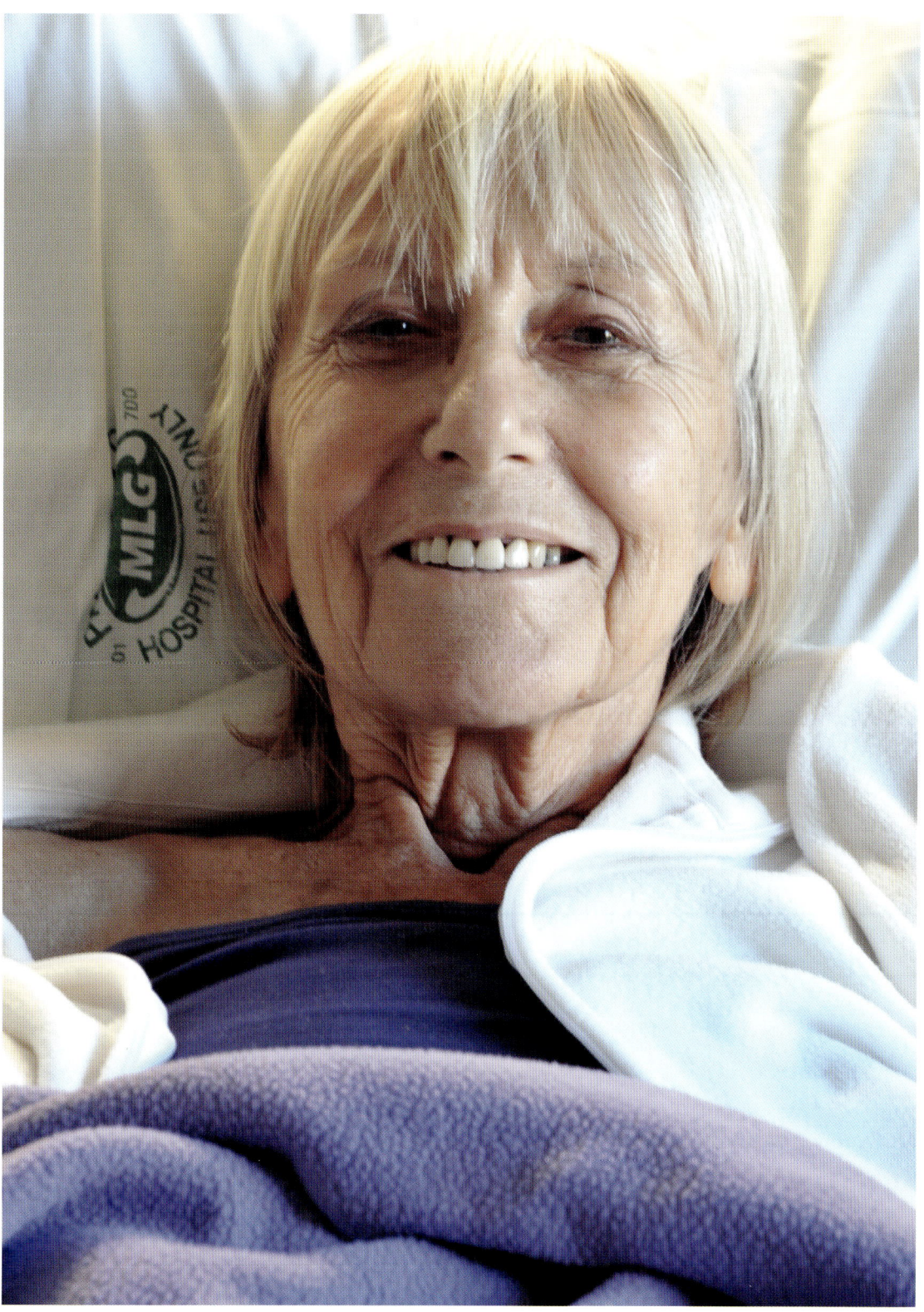

to get it for a second time. But that's life, or death, I suppose.

When I had my diagnosis this time, I kind of felt I knew it was coming. I used to do yoga, so I knew my body well. I sort of knew it. I was having some pains and I started to find out what it was. It took about six months to find out exactly what was wrong. I didn't feel poorly in myself, but I did have a lot of aches and pains.

I am a positive person, I try to be anyhow. I came here after having treatment in Hereford and Cheltenham. We knew that they could slow the pace of the cancer but not cure it. So I came here. You're not written off, here. There are interesting things to do. So, for instance, I started my photographic project, taking pictures of the people who come into my room. The staff are amazing, they are very good. I wanted to take their pictures because I have a passion for photography. About six or eight years ago, I did a degree in photography and then an MA in photography. I went to Hereford first and then down to Newport, which was very good. It was a terrific challenge. It was tough, believe me, it was tough. My final project was something about mirrors. I looked at the mirrors that people use outside their houses when they live on blind bends; they are the prominently curved mirrors. I found that if you went up close to them, the views you get are completely different from what you imagine you'll get. Some of the reflections you get are very beautiful. I was quite happy with it.

I had done a nightschool course in the 1970s in photography, which was great. I enjoyed that, it gave me an interest. But then I took to it again and really enjoyed it. So I've furthered that interest since I've been here. I just wanted to get a single photograph of the people who come into the room; it takes the subjects out of their professional context. My idea now is to get photographs of my neighbours, or get someone to help me with that. You know what Hereford's like. There are lots of little black and white houses out in the country. Well, ours is like that. It's a little cul-de-sac and we look after one another in a funny kind of way. There is a sense of community. It's not about being fond of people, there are people I don't really like. But there's a sense of being thrown together, of making a life with others.

Though I've had a wonderful career, I've always had other interests. I love horses, for instance. I had a couple of little ponies. I have two daughters, too: Zolita and Millie. Millie is a creative designer for an agency. She's a project manager. Zolita is a nurse. Zolita and I were very fond of horses though Millie is allergic to them. When David, my first husband, died, Millie was nine. The people who we lived close to gave us a horse. We were very lucky. We would just go and hack out. We had a little DIY livery near home, that's what we'd do. Then we moved to Hereford and we were able to have a nice time hacking out.

I'd like to talk a little about the hospice, too.

> 'There are interesting things to do. So, for instance, I started my photographic project, taking pictures of the people who come into my room.'

They offer a lot of practical help, both emotionally and physically. Even the views outside are beautiful. The amount of support we get is overwhelming, it's ridiculous, really. I wouldn't criticise it. It is remarkable. They are genuinely engaged and people feel that. It is superb. It's a full-on day, you don't get to sit and do nothing and get bored. There was a poetry session today, for instance. I do write poems, they are not great, but I write them. I have a book that somebody lent me, Liz Berry. She has an amazing voice. I've been sitting here trying to do her voice. I love poems. I taught A level English, so I had to really think about what people were saying, I couldn't just skim. I really enjoyed what people were saying and I became familiarised with what people were saying. All I can remember is Larkin saying: 'What will survive of us is love'. I'll probably get that carved for a seat.

I love novels, too. I'm very 19th century with novels. I loved Dickens. If you don't want a novel to end, read Dickens. It goes on forever.

When I look back over my life, I think about the things I've learned most. I love my parents. I sometimes wish I had been more emphatic in telling them how much I loved them. Both are dead now. But that's the main thing. Family is everything.

In My Room

St Michael's photography project by Ann Kay

Ann Kay was an inpatient at St Michael's Hospice for 12 weeks, during which time she created a collection of photographs.

The idea for the project came from a conversation with Hospice employee Chris Smart. Both were graduates of the Documentary Photography Course, at the University of The South Wales, in Newport.

While on the course, Ann had learned that great photographs were taken by photographers who had an insight into the subjects they were documenting. Ann wanted to show that people brought more than just their professional lives into her room. Ann's conversations with staff were about more than her health; they were about grandchildren, wedding plans, music and even honey. Ann wanted to show the humanity behind the uniforms worn by staff. After an informal chat; Ann asked each of her subjects to choose a prop to be photographed with that was significant in their life.

Ann said: "I don't know what I would have done without this project, it helped me to feel brighter in myself. Photography is something that I enjoy and working on the project kept me busy. Creating these photographs has been about living every moment of my life. I hope that one day these pictures will be in an exhibition."

The photographs were all taken during Ann's stay, and although Chris was needed to press the button, Ann directed the shoot. She gave instructions about how to get the best visual effect, and she used her wit to engage with her subjects. As the shoot progressed, Chris would show Ann the pictures, and she would ask for alterations until she approved each shot. Chris then printed out an A3 photograph and displayed it in Ann's room. The images created a buzz in the unit, among Ann's guests and members of staff. The portraits stimulated new conversations between a spectrum of people about the big and the small things in life. The captions that accompany the pictures on the following pages are Ann's words.

Ann died on 28th December 2015 after spending 12 weeks at St Michael's. Chris and Ann's family hope her photographs will stimulate more conversations about the work of St Michael's staff, who give people the chance to live every moment of life.

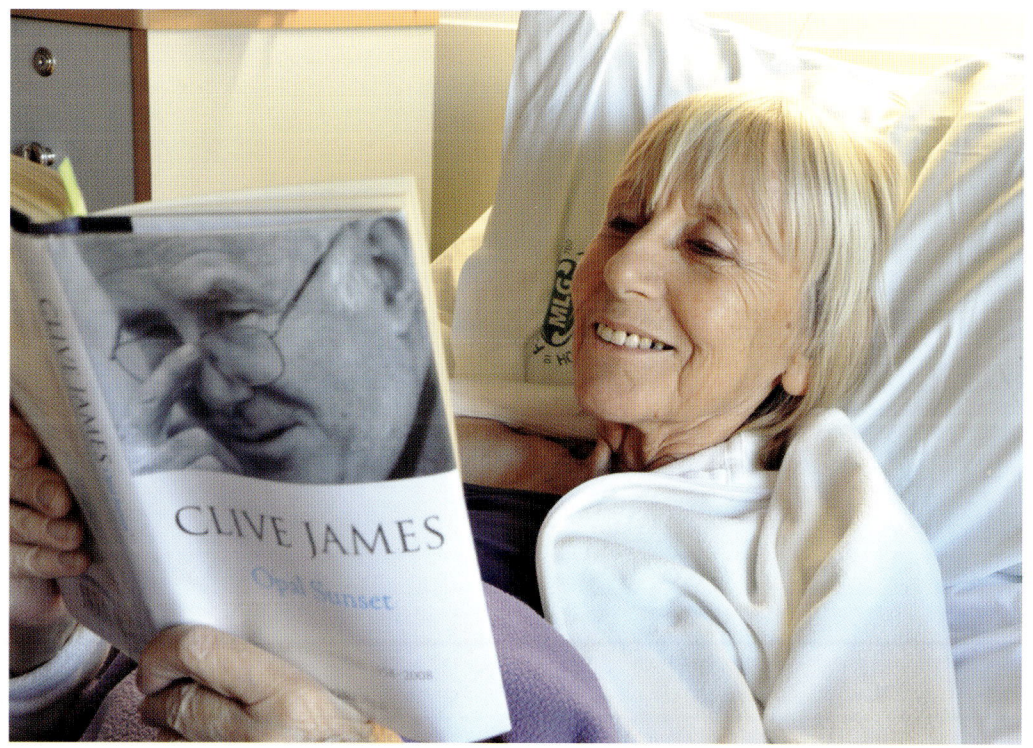

In My Room

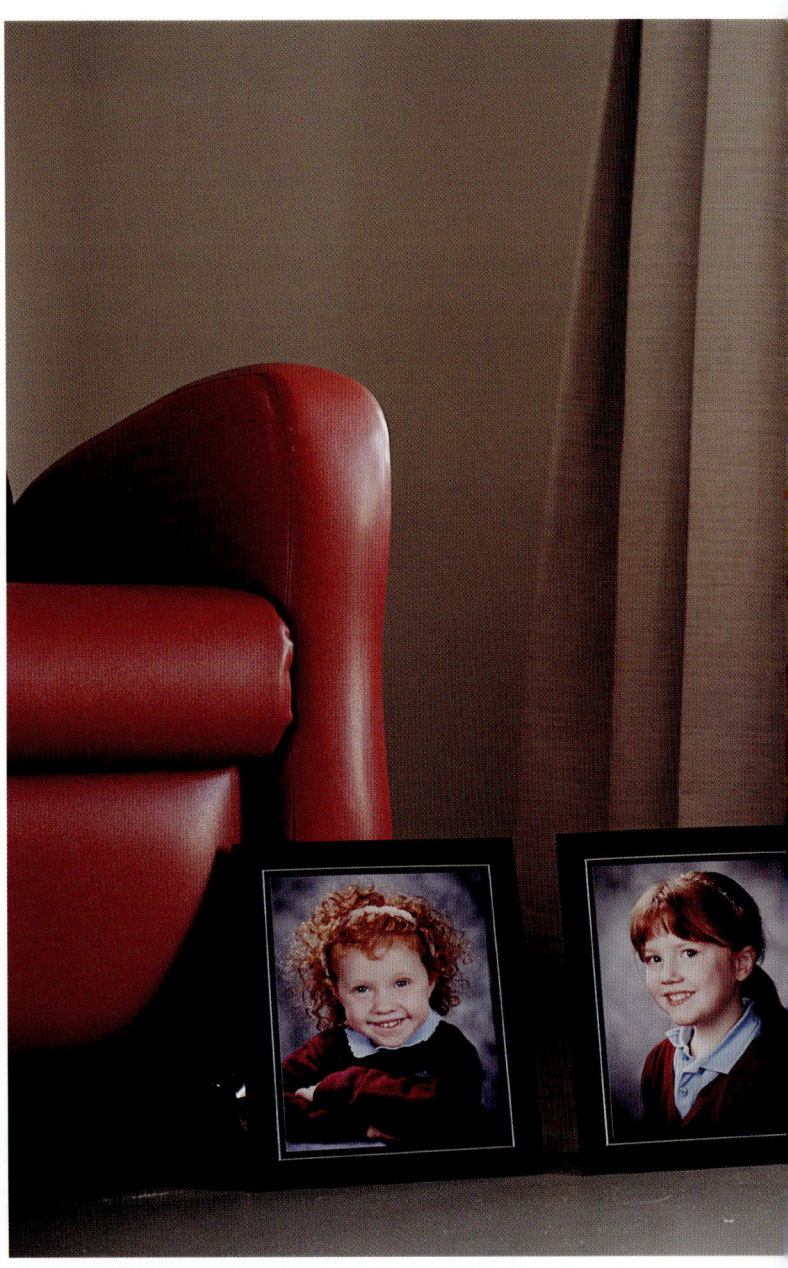

Helen has been a constant presence in the room and takes great care about prescribing the right medication. She will talk to me about running and her children but only when I ask and I appreciate that.

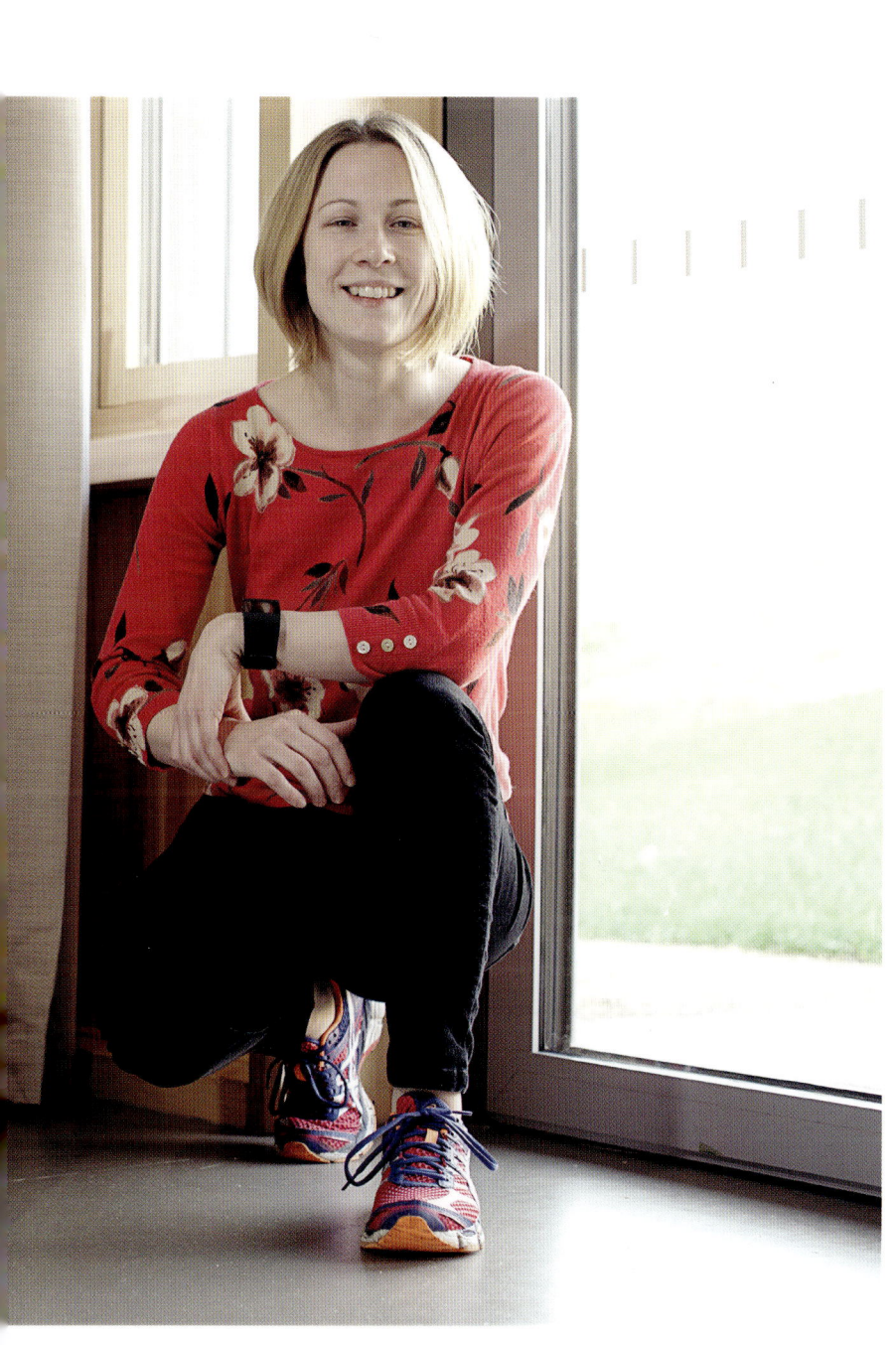

In My Room

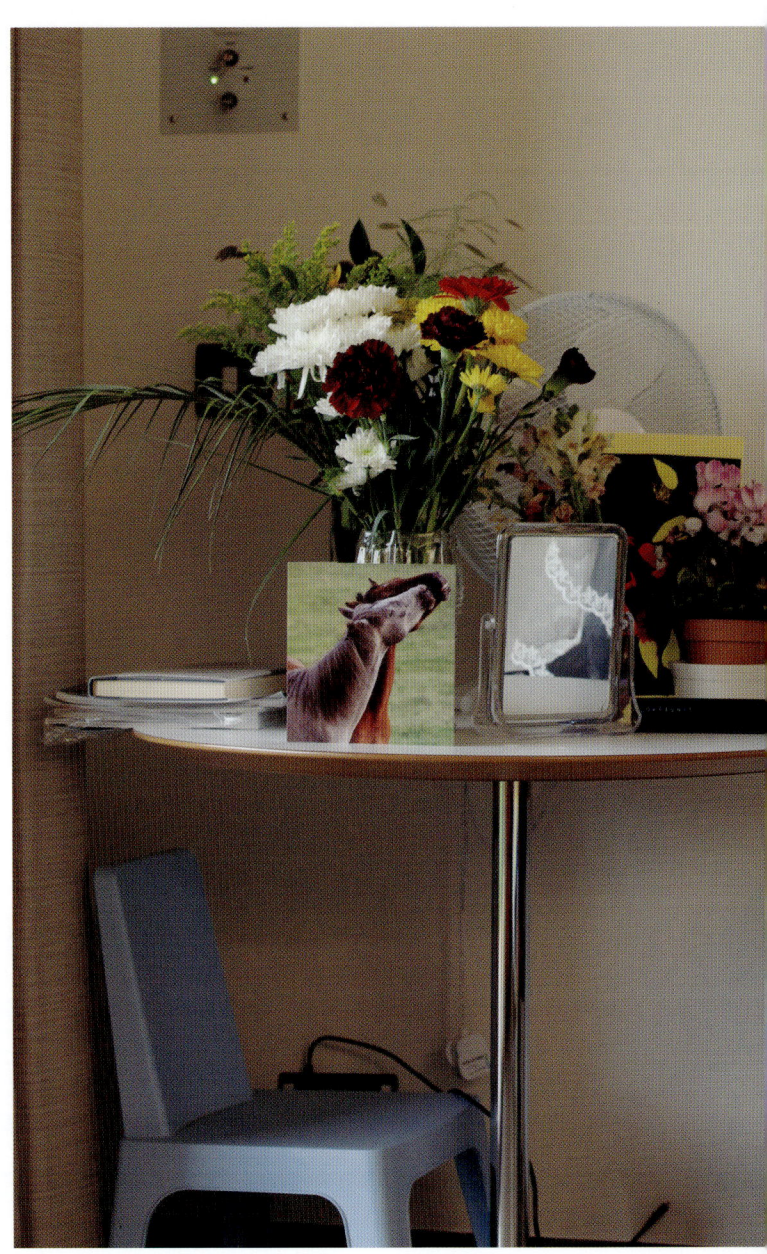

Jade's Madonna-like face and slender figure made her an exceptional bride the week after this photograph was taken. She has so much depth to her personality. She works very hard for the hospice.

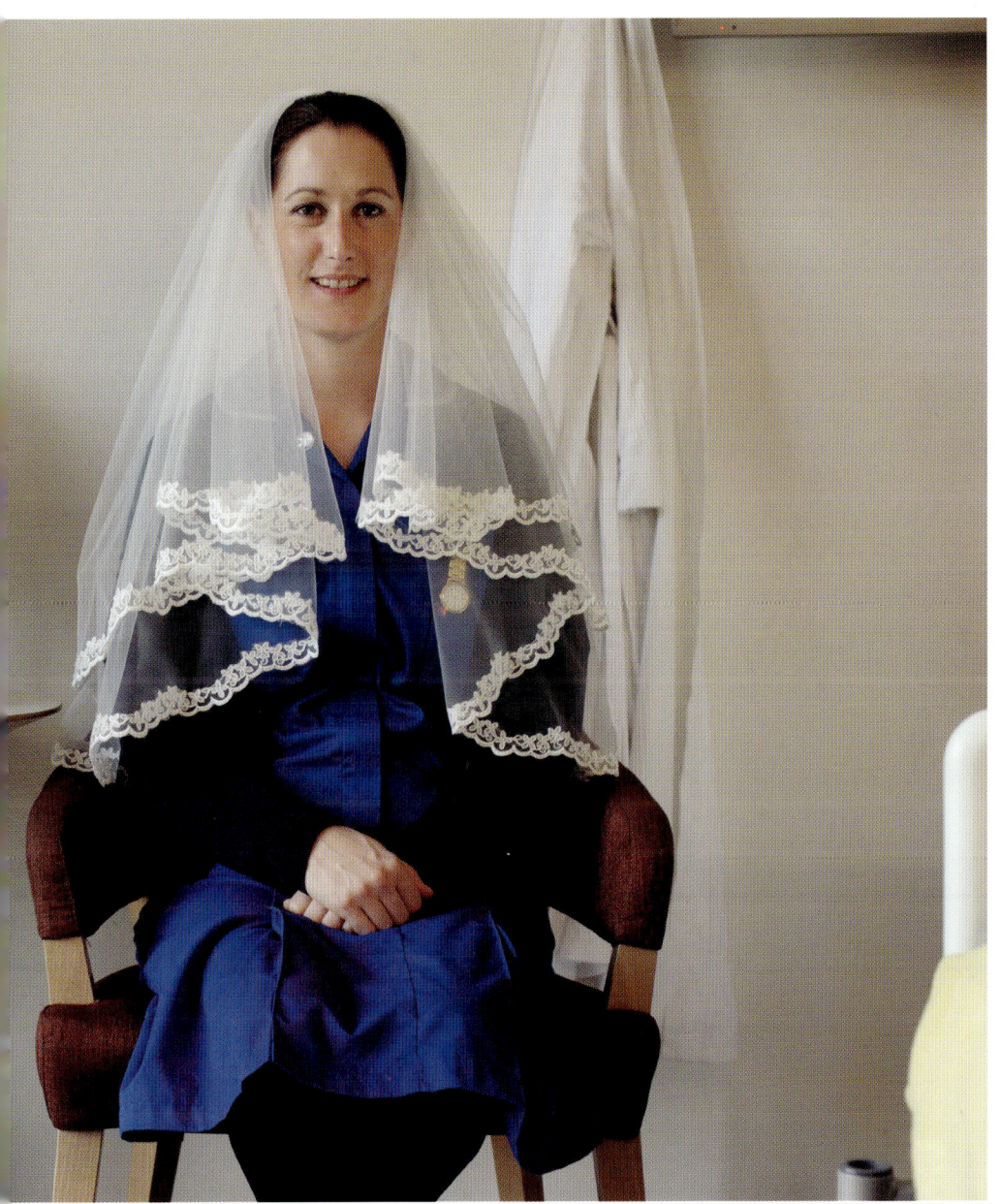

In My Room

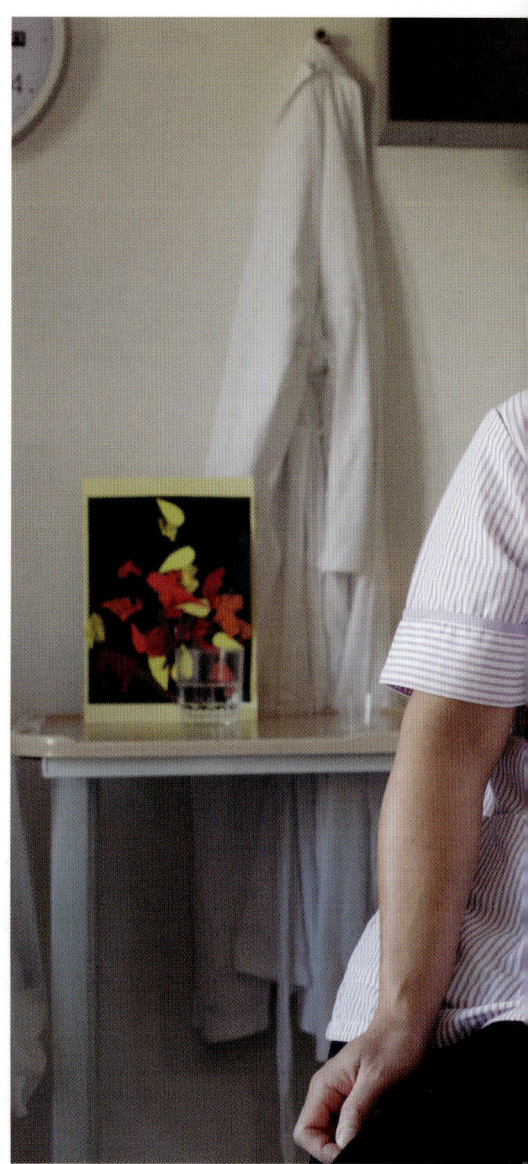

Parti's son was rescued by the Air Ambulance service after a road traffic accident. Working at St Michael's helps her live with that memory and enables her to give something back to humanity. She's hilarious but underneath it all she is dedicated to helping the hospice survive and prosper.

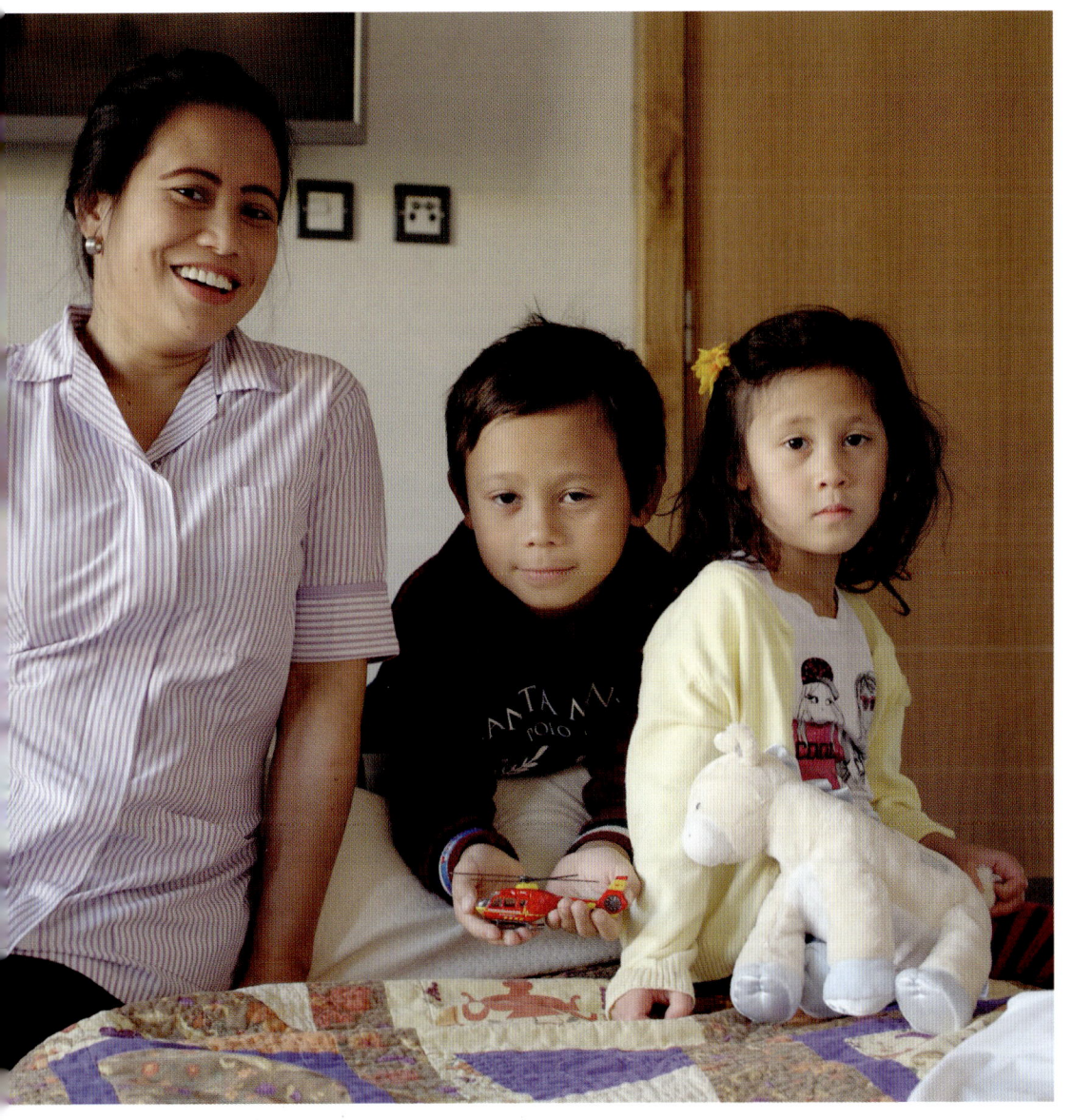

In My Room

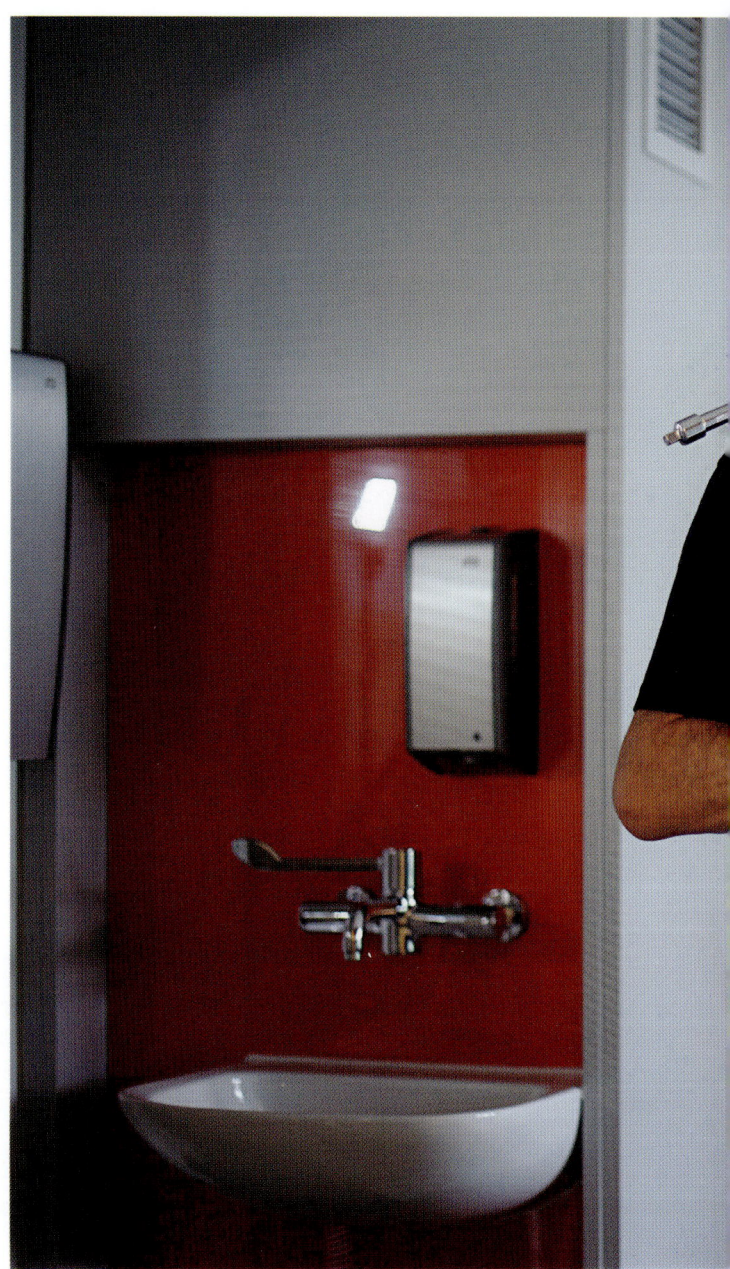

Keith loves to fix things. While he was unblocking the sink, I saw that he has a real rapport with Parti. It's good to watch. Together they reveal something more about the hospice and the relaxed and pleasant atmosphere.

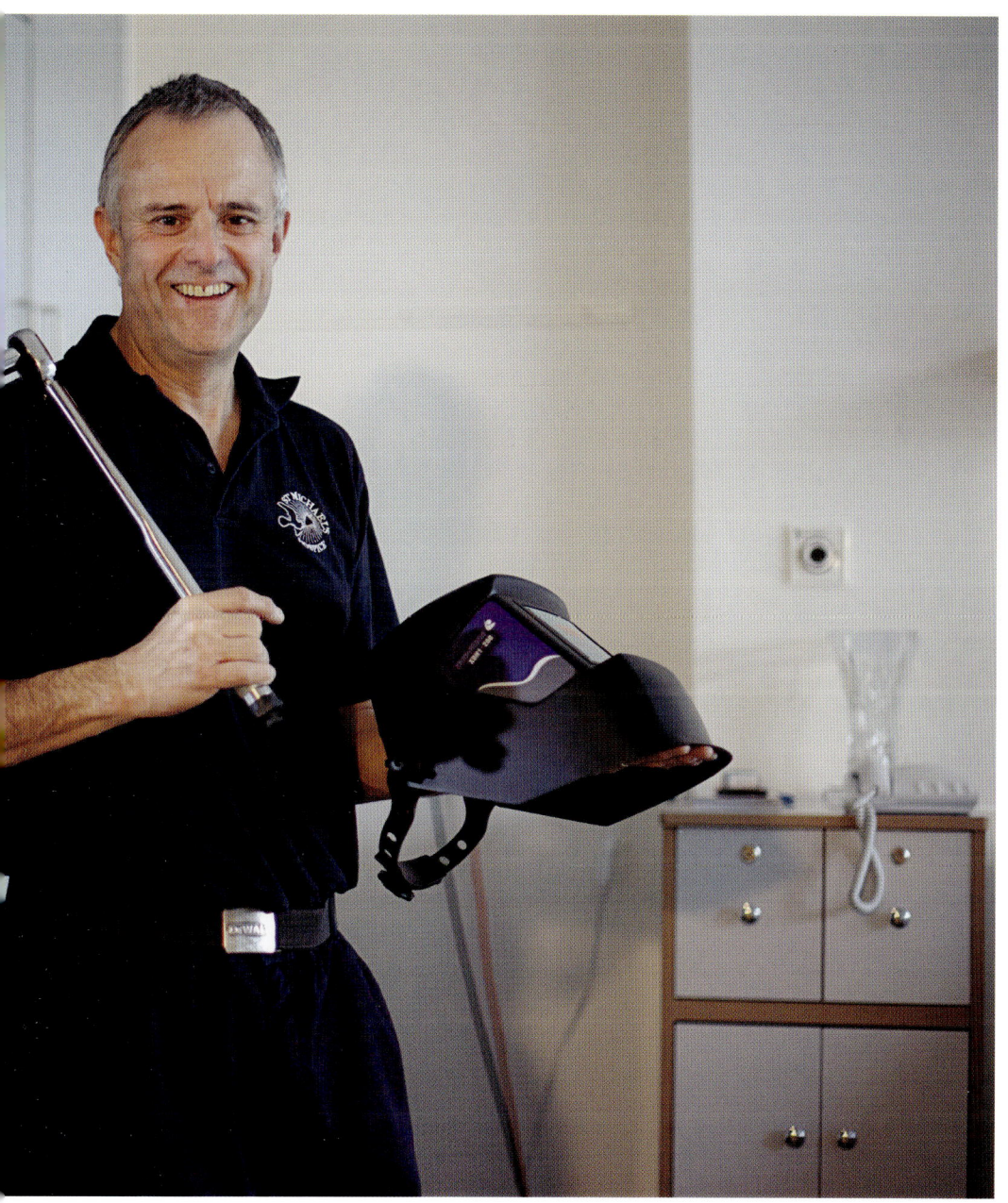

In My Room

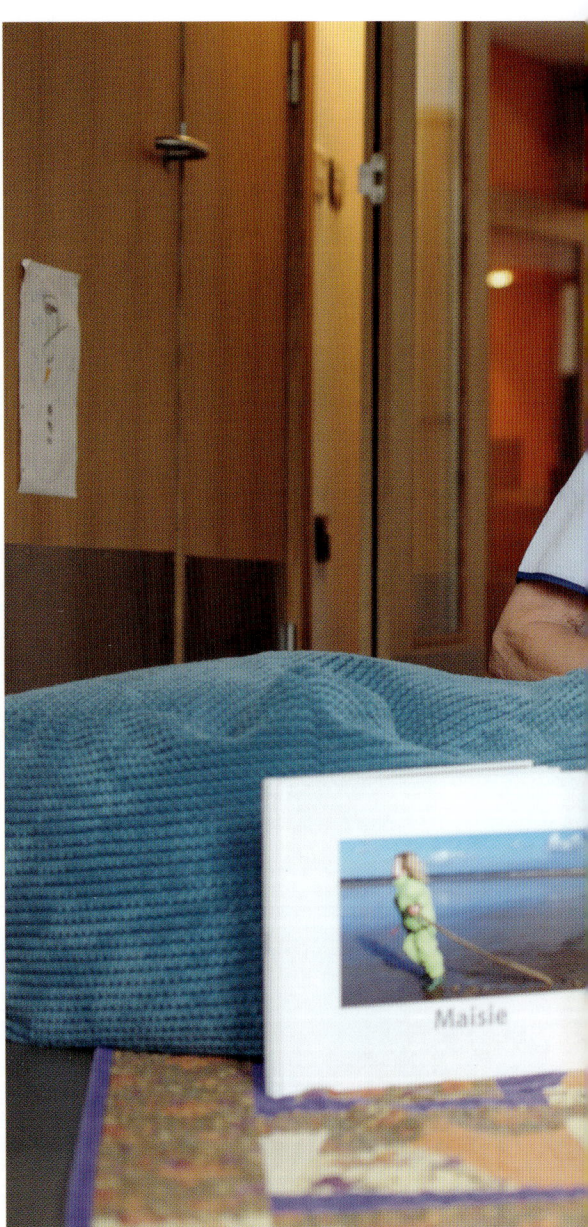

Margaret brings light into the room. She works quietly and with great compassion. We are very different, but she connected with me in same the way I connected with her. She is a shining example of how a grandmother can be.

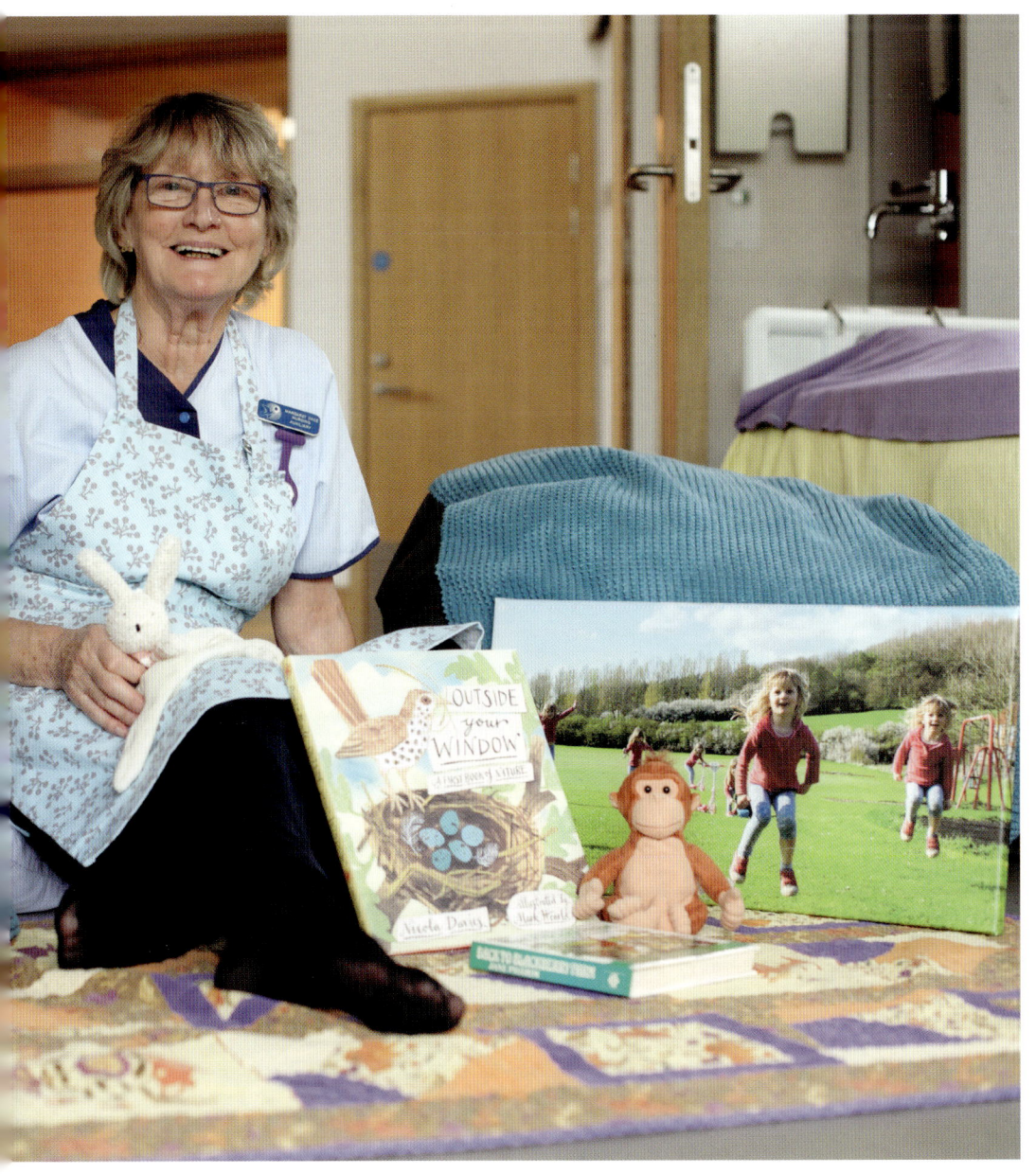

In My Room

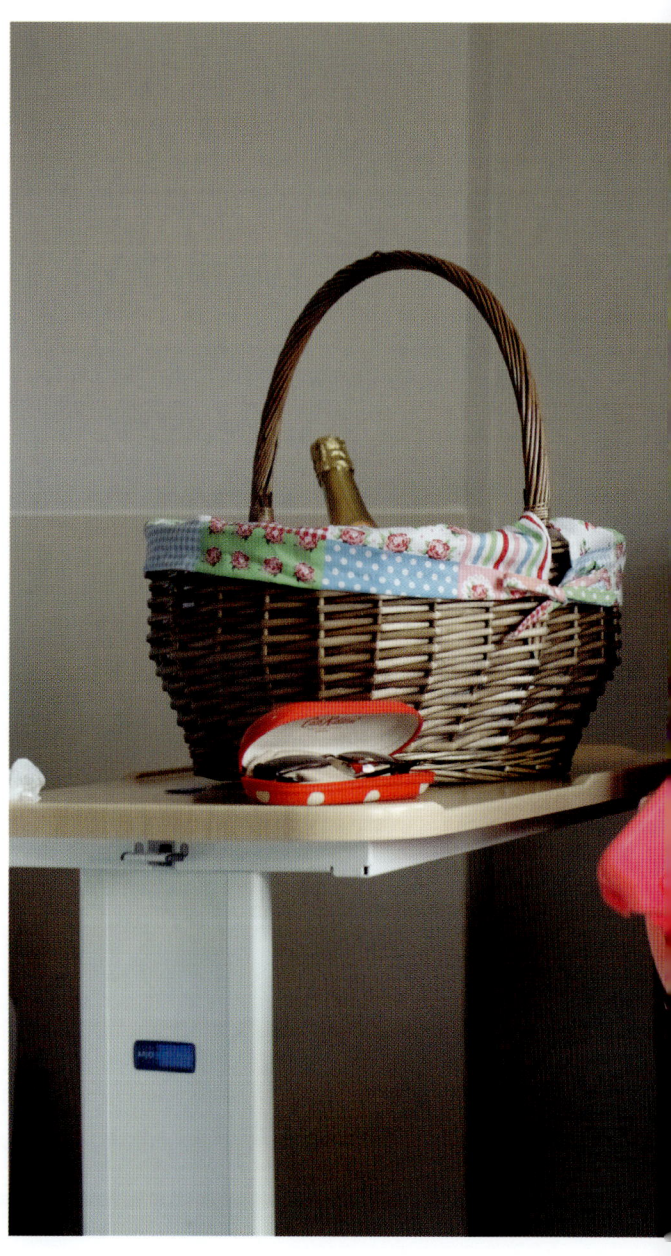

Nikki comes and asks very kindly what I want to eat. I haven't got an appetite for anything, but she keeps coming, and she keeps asking. I appreciate her determination to deliver the highest quality of care.

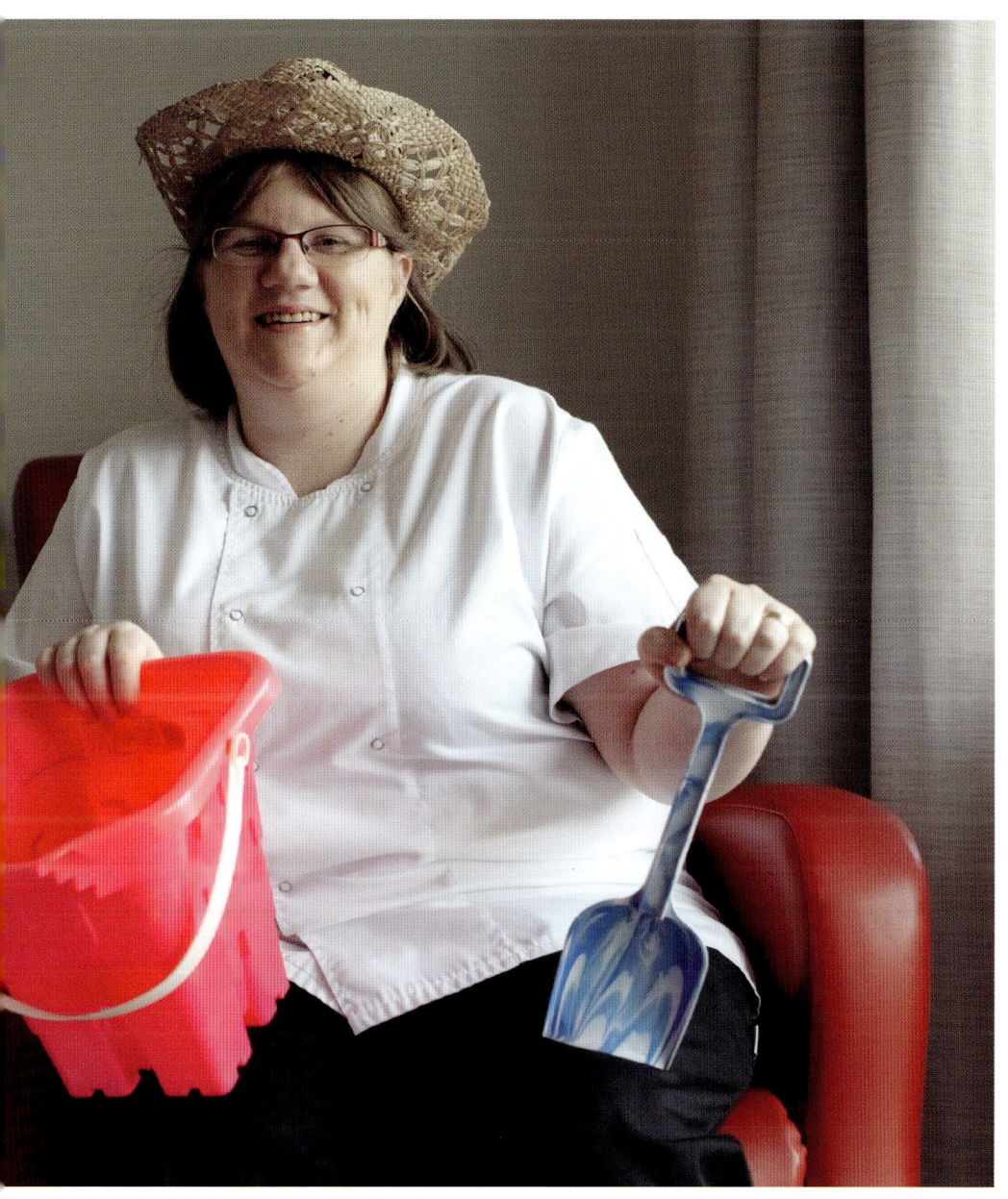

In My Room

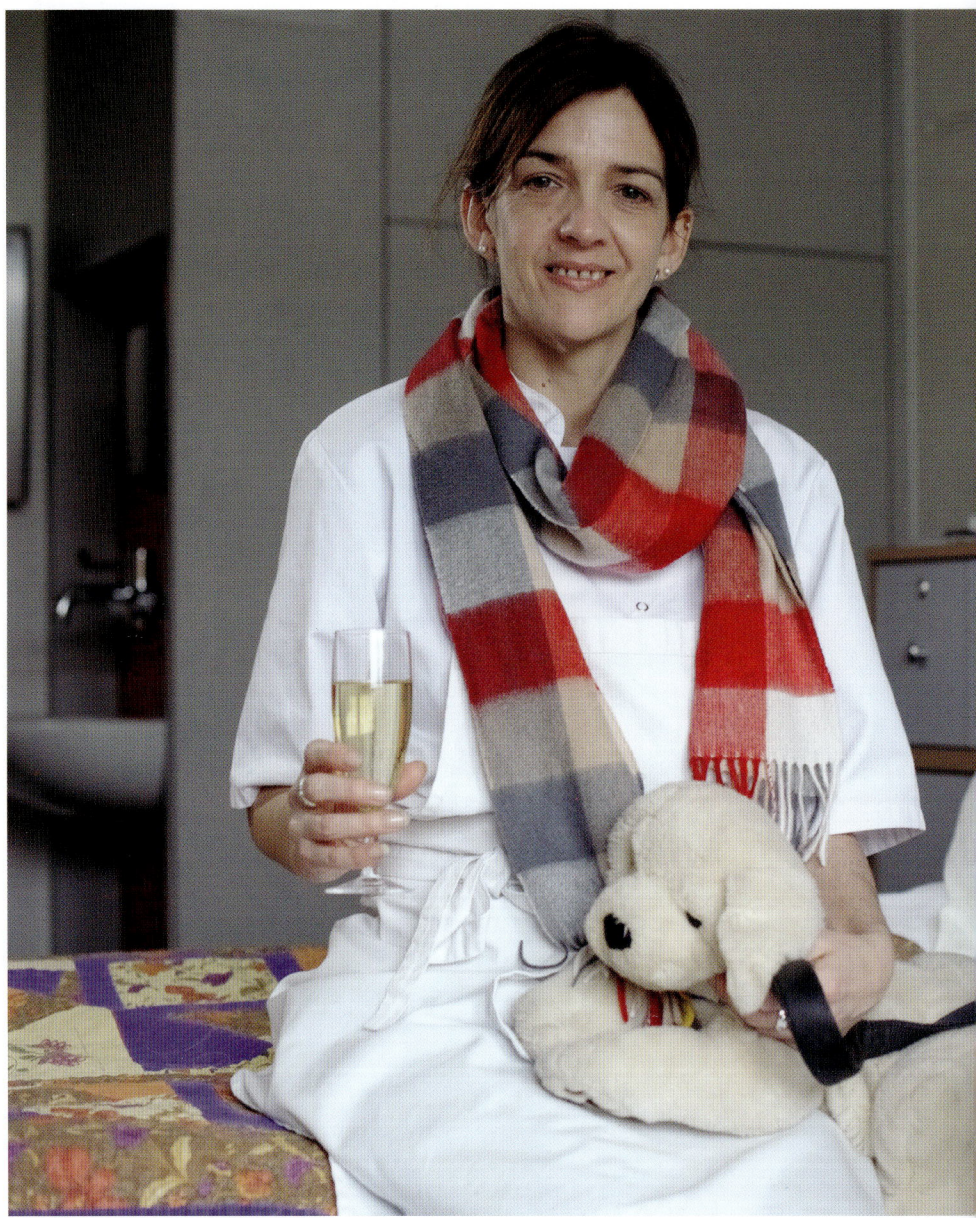

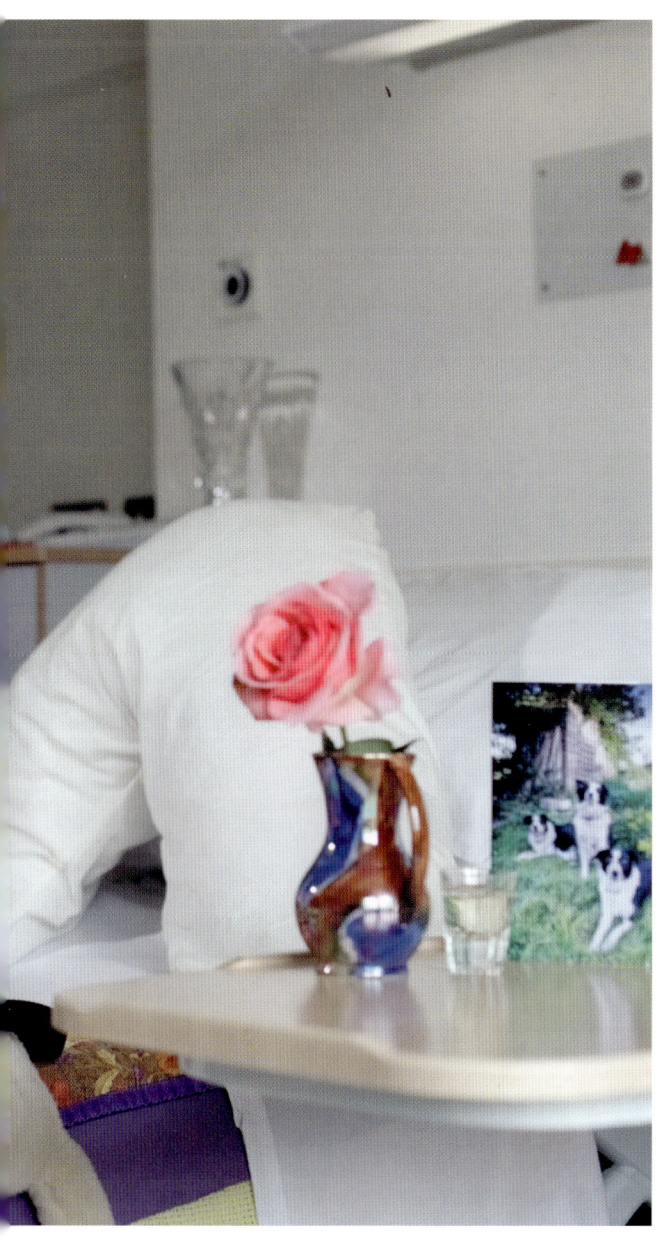

Rachel is an extremely gentle person. Her daughter works here too, she is as gentle as her mother. Rachel's face is a symbol of goodness. She gets a lot of enjoyment from knowing how much people benefit from the good food she prepares.

In My Room

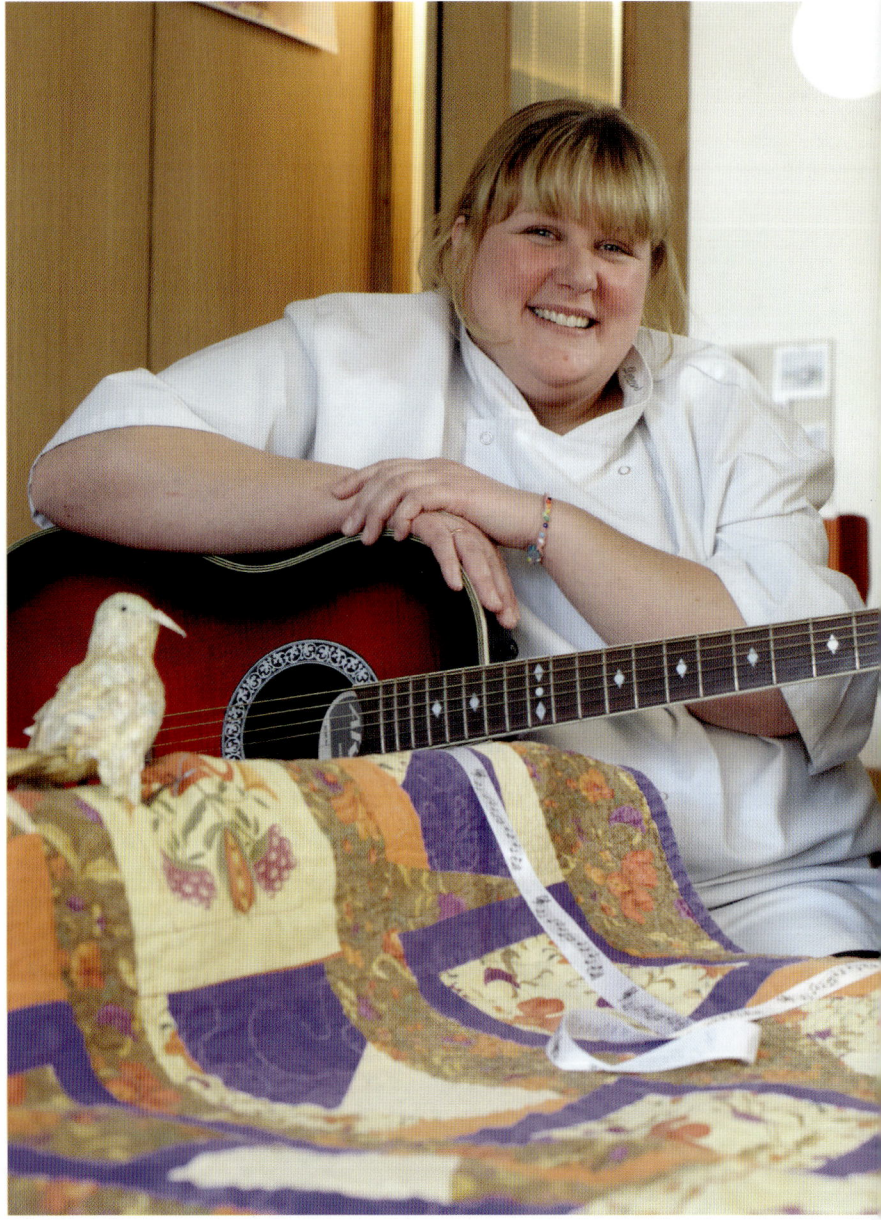

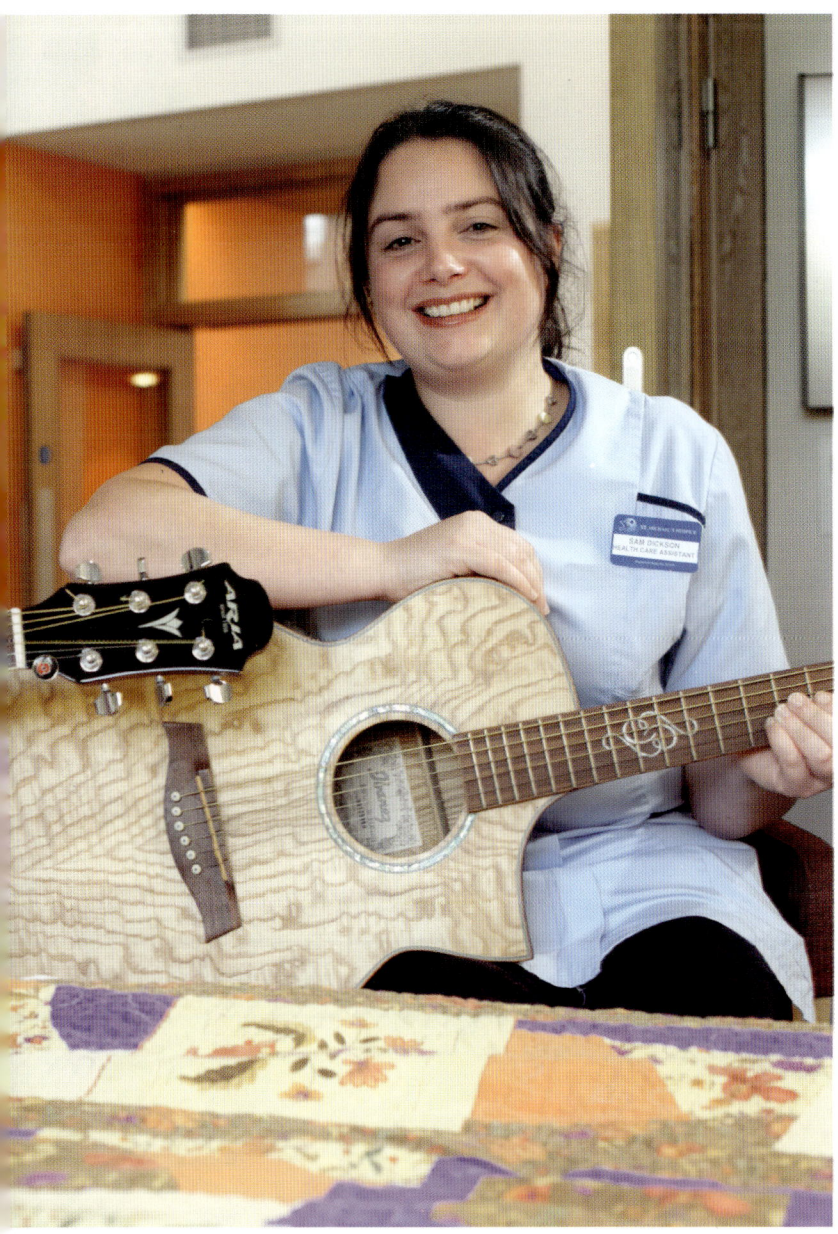

Both Sam and Collette have bright open faces. They bring their youthfulness to
the work they do. They wanted to come and play their instruments and I was
very happy to listen. So we all played our parts. It was so interesting to hear
hymns played in a completely different way.

In My Room

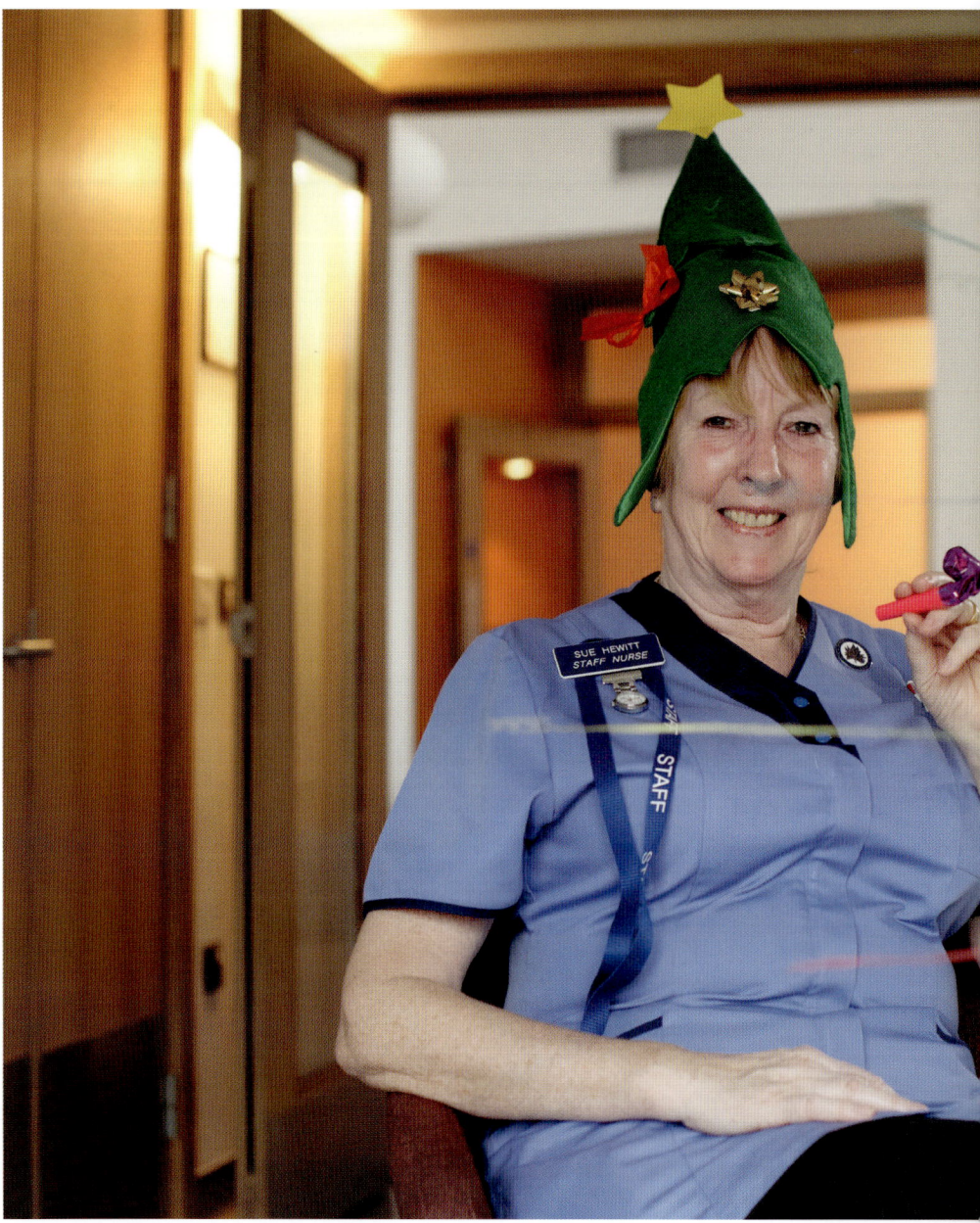

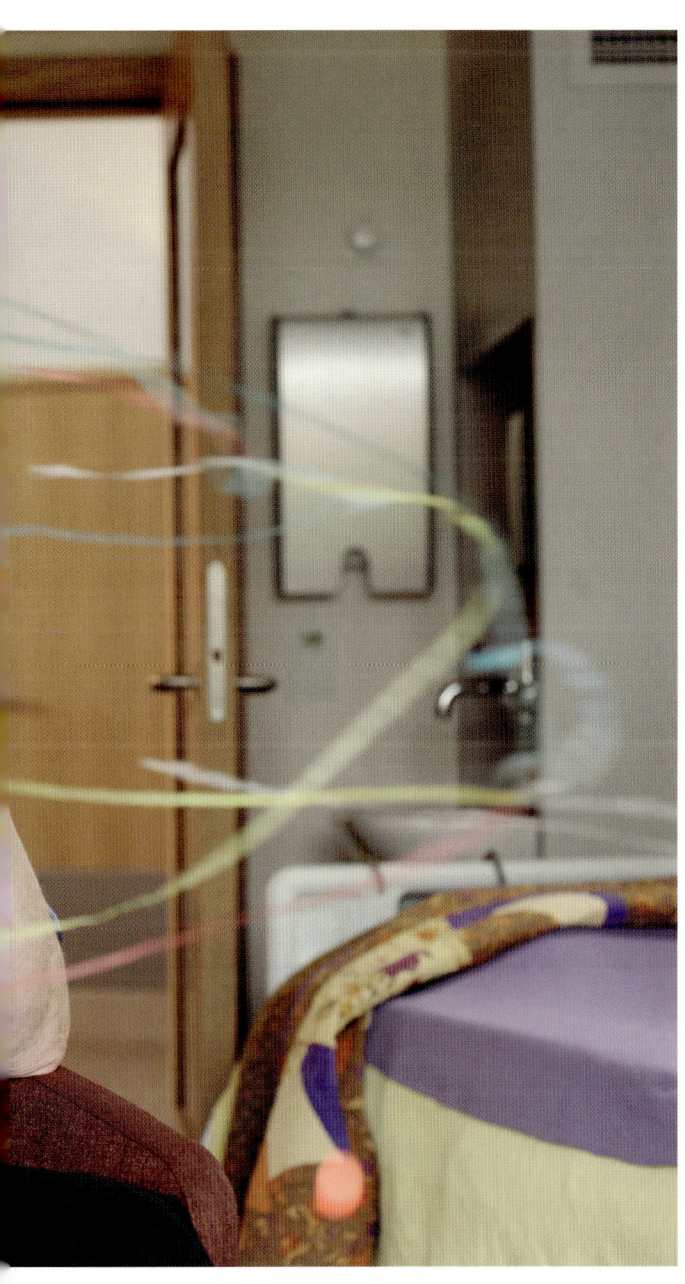

Sue has told me about a letter she received from a patient's husband. He thanked her for all she had done in lifting the mood when his wife was at St Michaels.

In My Room

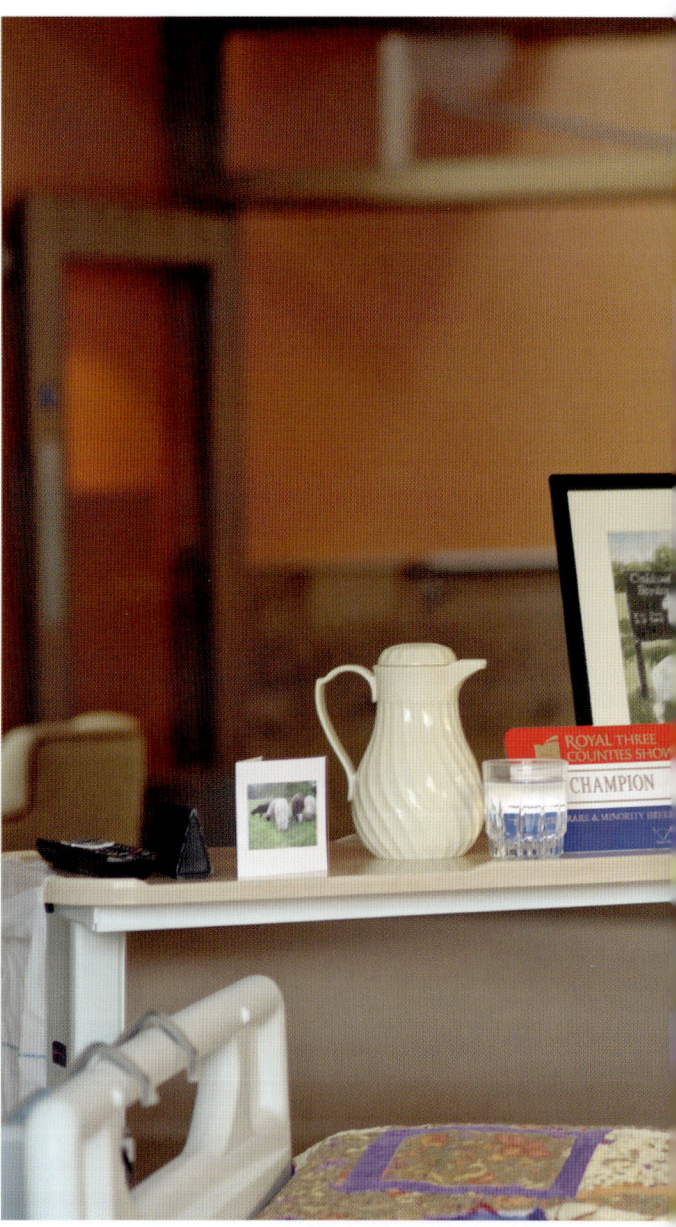

Lorna brings laughter into the room. She works hard and with real compassion and has fun too. She is most proud of her son. He's an award-winning shepherd, and has achieved all this at the age of 16.

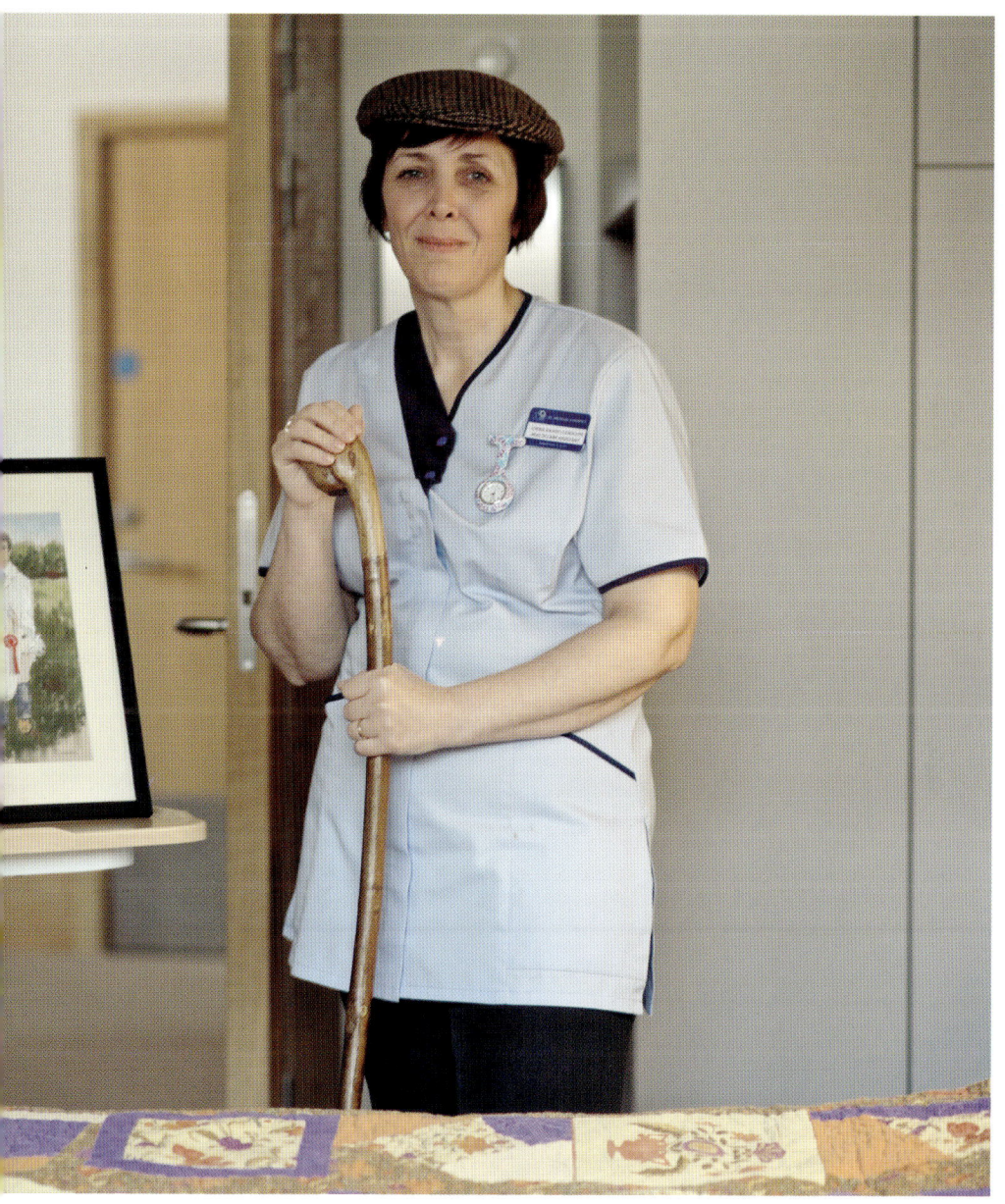

In My Room

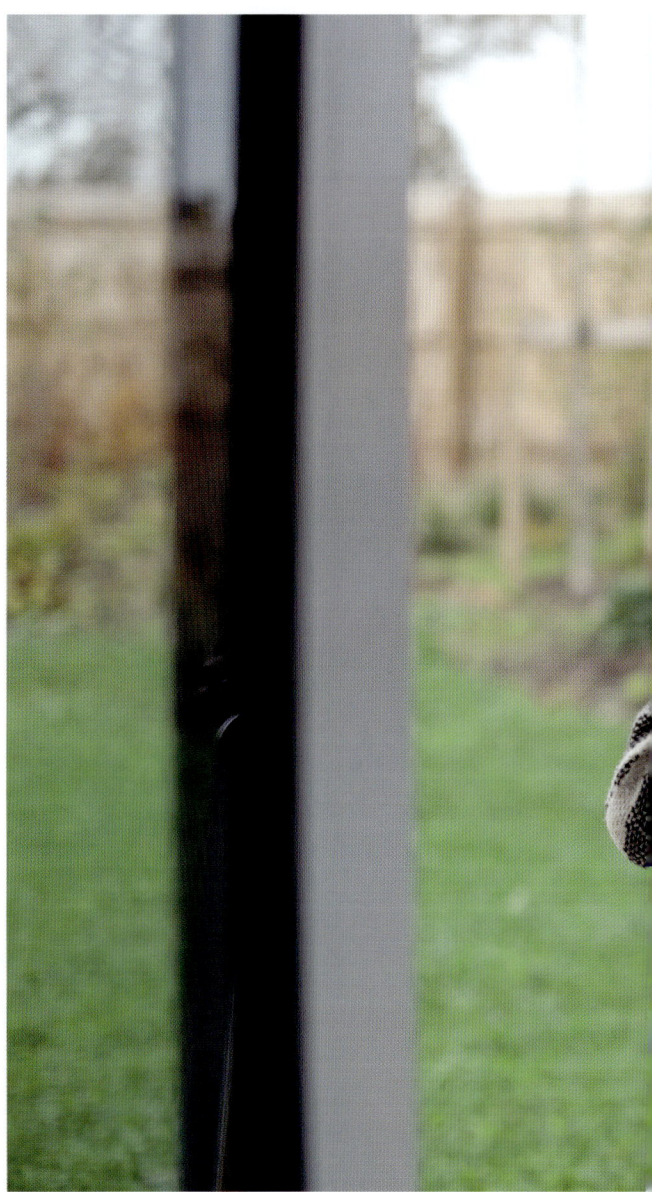

Mary helps people overcome the problems they face when they or someone they love are diagnosed with a terminal illness. She's gently relentless to ensure everyone is supported in the right way. Mary's other passion is organising the Three Choirs Fringe Festival.

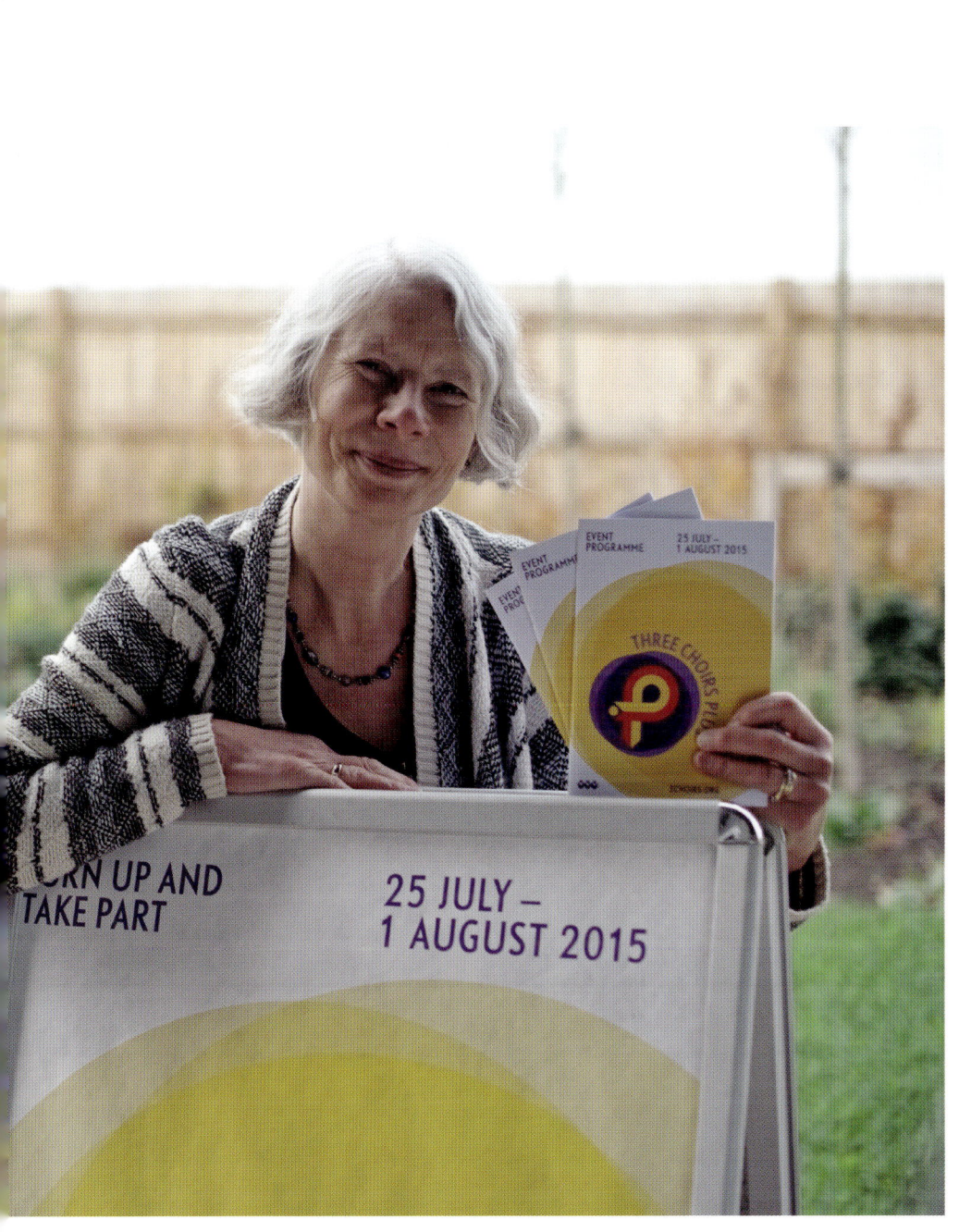

In My Room

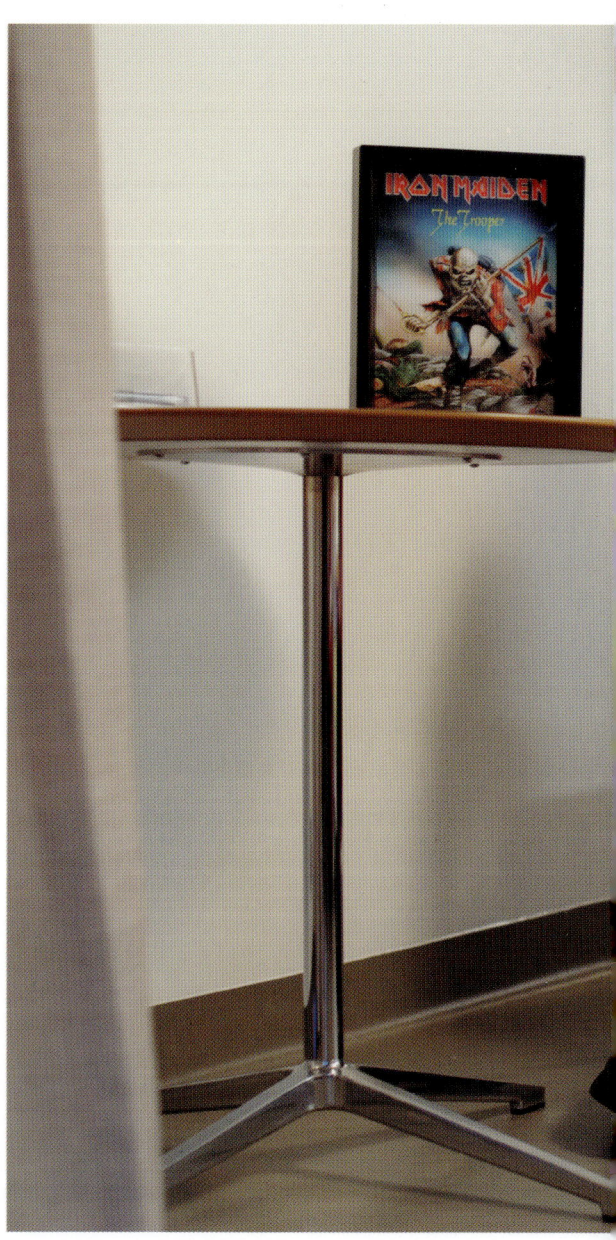

Tash is like Florence Nightingale, dedicated to looking after her patients. When she's not on duty, she puts on her leather boots and becomes an Iron Maiden. She is the proud owner of one of Iron Maiden's Nicko McBrain's drumsticks, which she caught in a scrum.

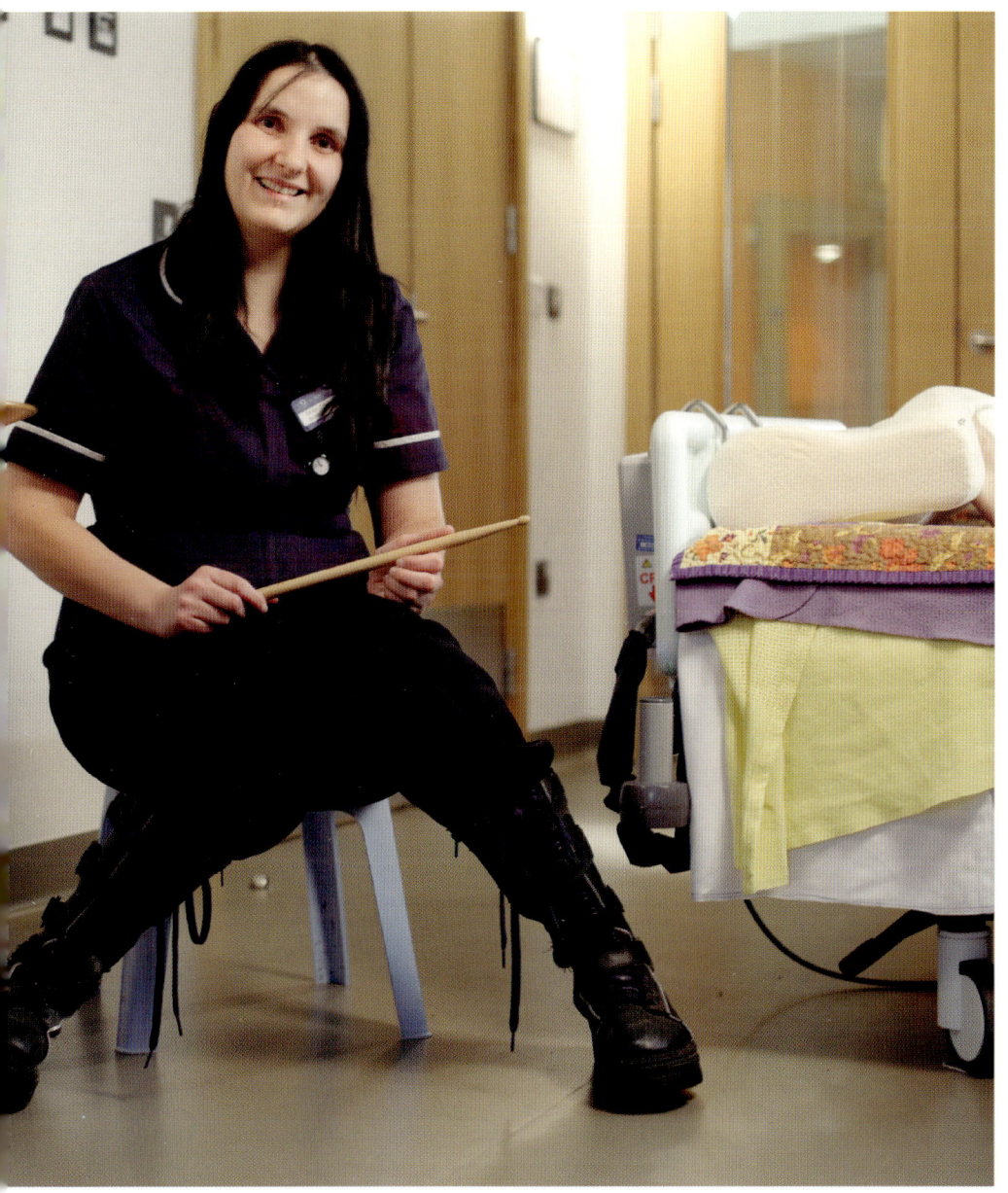

In My Room

I imagine Tony talks as gently to his bees
as he does to his patients. He brings a
feeling of milk and honey into the room.
He knows that being a doctor is not just
about what's written in the medical books.
He knows it's about understanding that
patients need to be treated with respect
and dignity.

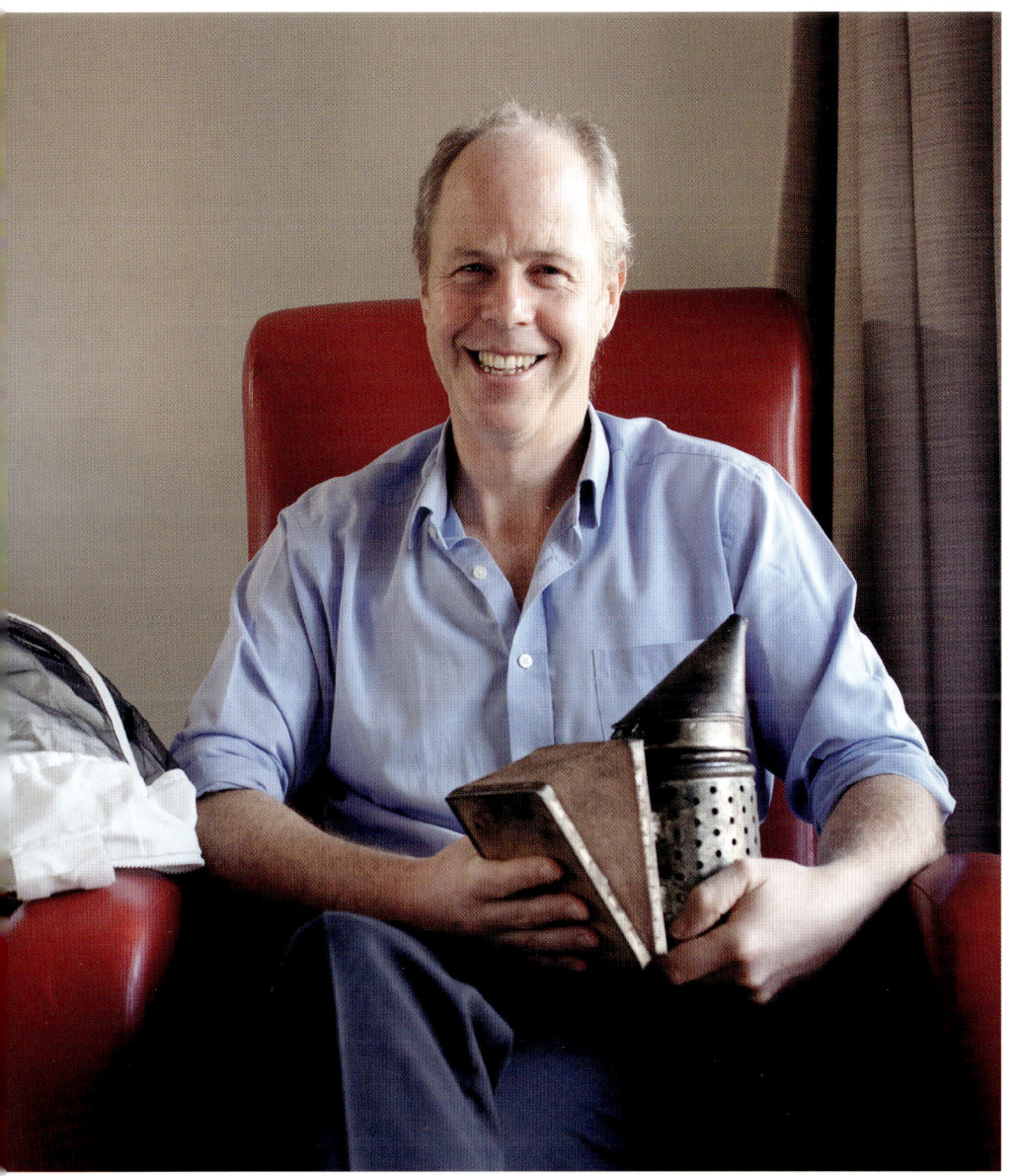

DONATE TODAY

St Michael's Hospice relies on donations. And you can help us make life better for patients and their loved ones living with a life-limiting illness.

We want to help people to live well until the end of life, and we want to continue supporting their friends and families for as long as they need us. We can only continue providing our quality clinical care, free of charge, to all the people who need it if we have your support.

It costs £4.6million every year to run St Michael's Hospice and 90 pence out of every £1 spent on care comes from voluntary donations. Because of you, and the thousands of other generous people who have given their time, money and support, St Michael's Hospice can continue to be a place of light and love.

By donating today, you will make an immediate difference to the people we care for, now and for future generations. Everyone has the right to die with dignity and support; your donation, whatever the size, makes it possible for us to provide that support and care.

Making a regular donation will help us continue to provide a complete end-of-life care service free of charge.

When someone we love dies, it can also help to do something positive in their memory.

For many families whose loved one received care at St Michael's Hospice, making a donation in their name is a way of celebrating their life. For others, it can seem like an appropriate way of saying thank you, or of giving something back.

Many families ask for donations instead of flowers at a funeral, and we can help by providing donation envelopes. The envelopes also mean taxpayers can Gift Aid their donation. Collection tins and buckets are also available.

Whatever your reason, any donation, no matter how big or small, will be gratefully received. Your gift will ensure St Michael's Hospice can continue providing love and care to other patients and their families for generations to come.

Giving in memory can be something you do once, or on a long-term basis. Many families set up a Tribute Fund in a loved one's name.

Making a significant personal donation or giving through your own Trust or Foundation makes a real difference to your local community.

To help St Michael's meet this challenge, we are asking people to join with other philanthropic benefactors and ensure St Michael's Hospice continues to be a place of light and love for generations to come.

People give large donations for many different reasons and we always want to listen to the stories that have inspired such enormous generosity. In return for your gift, we will do whatever we can to give you something back. By listening to you, we will do our utmost to find an appropriate way of showing recognition for the difference you make to all of us.

Thank you from all of us for your generosity.

Thanks to:

Russell
Dotty
Fiona
John
Marian and Dennis
Christine
Geraldine
Mur
Rhyanne
Mike
Ann
Brian
Ethel
Jade
Janet
Cicely and Cyril
Pam
Terry
Tessa and Ken
Ann – for inspiration, hope and a sense of perspective

Further thanks to:

Ruth Denison – for patience and steely determination in bringing the project to life

Rachel Shortt – for helping to ensure the legacy of the patients featured in 20 Beds

Chris Smart – for his work on In My Room

Nicky West – for support and encouragement

Rachel Haworth – for being on board from the off and for suggesting the title

Andy Cooke – for boundless enthusiasm and optimism

Carl Jones – for a beautifully-written history

David Briggs – for efficiency, diligence and creative design

All patients, staff, volunteers, friends and supporters of St Michael's Hospice, present and past